MCQs on Microbial Diseases in Veterinary Medicine

MCQs on Microbial Diseases in Veterinary Medicine

By :

S. SARAVANAN

Assistant Professor
Department of Veterinary Epidemiology and
Preventive Medicine
Veterinary College and Research Institutes
Namakkal-637 002, Tamil Nadu (India)

SSPH

SATISH SERIAL PUBLISHING HOUSE

403, Express Tower, Commercial Complex, Azadpur, Delhi-110033 (India)
Phone : 011-27672852, Fax : 91-11-27672046
E-mail : info@satishserial.com, hkjain1975@yahoo.com
Website : www.satishserial.com

Published by :

SATISH SERIAL PUBLISHING HOUSE

403, Express Tower, Commercial Complex, Azadpur, Delhi-110033 (INDIA)
Phone : 011-27672852 Fax : 91-11-27672046
E-mail : info@satishserial.com, hkjain1975@yahoo.com

ISBN 978-93-84053-12-3

Typeset at: Harminder Kharb *for* Laxmi Art Creation
Printed at: Salasar Imaging Systems, Delhi-110035

PREFACE

The book being an examination guide to students, presents *multiple choice questions* (MCQ) in Veterinary Medicine on various infectious diseases of bacterial, viral, rickettsial, chlamydial and fungal origin in livestock and poultry, with solved answers. It covers all the facets of a disease like various synonyms, epidemiology, pathogenesis and clinical signs, prevention and control including disinfection, latest trends in vaccination, etc. in the setting of questions.

I hope, certainly, this book might cater to the thirst of zealous students holding the B.V.Sc. & A. H. or M.V.Sc. degree in Veterinary Medicine or Preventive Medicine or Veterinary Microbiology and make the graduates keep abreast of various key answers related to various microbial infections in the above fields. Perusal of this question bank might definitely increase the thinking and answering ability of the students and make them hassle free before appearing in the regular under graduate examinations (as per VCI curriculum), Public Service Examinations and other Competitive examinations as well which assess the performance of the students or graduates based on their ability to select the correct answer in MCQ. In this book, questions are presented in a shuffled manner, not categorized into various chapters like bacterial diseases, viral diseases etc., as this could narrow down the answering ability of the students within the selected area (chapter).

In this question bank, since the answers are paged last, the students are requested to analyse the answers with ample time patiently, choose out the right or best answer leaving out ambiguous ones and finally evaluate themselves after reading out key answers in the last page.

I wish the aspiring students for all success in their career.

Author

CONTENTS

MCQs on Microbial Diseases in Veterinary Medicine

1. *C. pseudotuberculosis* can affect
   a) Sheep and goat b) Cattle
   c) Man d) All of the above

2. The bacteria *C. pseudotuberculosis* is
   a) Gram negative b) Capsule forming
   c) Motile d) None of the above

3. Ulcerative lymphangitis is primarily a disease of
   a) Horses b) Sheep
   c) Goats d) All of the above

4. Which one of the following is not a method of transmission in horses?
   a) Ingestion b) Inhalation
   c) Direct contact d) Arthropod bite

5. Percutaneous transmission of *Strongyloides westeri* favours the transmission of
   a) Ulcerative lymphangitis b) Glanders
   c) Strangles d) Equine encephalitis

6. Which one of the following is a disinfectant of choice in the control of anthrax?
   a) 5% Phenol b) 5% Sodium hydroxide
   c) 10% -20% formalin d) All the above

7. Which one of the following is favorable for anthrax outbreak?
   a) >15°C and >95 Rh b) <15°C and <95 Rh
   c) >15°C and <95 Rh d) <15°C and >95 Rh

8. Anthrax is more common in
   a) Cattle and sheep b) Sheep and goat
   c) Horse d) Cattle and buffalo

9. Anthrax is transmitted among animals mostly by
   a) Ingestion b) Inhalation
   c) Skin penetration d) Arthropod bite

10. Cutaneous anthrax is common in the following
    a) Cattle b) Sheep
    c) Pig d) Man

11. Which one of the following is most susceptible to infection by *M.bovis*?
    a) Horse b) Sheep
    c) Pig d) Man

12. Ingestion is the method of transmission of tuberculosis in
    a) Cattle b) Sheep
    c) Pig d) Man

13. Cell mediated immune response is important for acquired resistance against the following disease
    a) Tuberculosis b) Brucellosis
    c) Rinderpest d) All the above

14. The effective eradication method in tuberculosis is
    a) Test and slaughter policy b) Vaccination
    c) Isolation d) Seromonitoring

15. Which one of the following type of tubercle bacilli commonly affects human?
    a) Vole type b) Bovine type
    c) Avian type d) All the above

16. The following are the risk factors for the incidence of clinical paratuberculosis
    a) Parturition b) Acidity of the soil
    c) Overcrowding d) All the above

17. The primary site of multiplication of bacilli in paratuberculosis is
    a) Small intestine
    b) Terminal part large intestine
    c) Terminal part of small and large intestine
    d) Jejunum

18. The following is the characteristic feature in sheep affected with Johne's disease
    a) Emaciation
    b) Diarrhoea
    c) Both of the above
    d) None of the above

19. The histotoxic clostridium is
    a) *Clostridium chauvoi*
    b) *Clostridium septicum*
    c) *Clostridium novy type A*
    d) All the above

20. Classical enterotoxaemia in ruminants is caused by
    a) *Clostridium perfringens type A*
    b) *Clostridium perfringens type B*
    c) *Clostridium perfringens type C*
    d) *Clostridium perfringens type D*

21. Malignant edema in sheep is caused by
    a) *Clostridium novy type A*
    b) *Clostridium novy type B*
    c) *Clostridium septicum*
    d) *Clostridium novy type D*

22. The lethal and necrotizing toxin causing classical enterotoxaemia is
    a) Alpha
    b) Epsilon
    c) Iota
    d) Enterotoxin

23. The risk factor responsible for enterotoxaemia is
    a) High rain fall
    b) Grazing on lush pasture
    c) Heavy grain feeding
    d) All the above

24. Which one of the following is not true for *C. tetani*?
    a) It exists in soil and manure
    b) Faecal material of man and horses are secondary habitat.
    c) It is non-saprophytic
    d) It is confined to alkaline and calcareous soil.

25. The most susceptible host for tetanus is
    a) Sheep b) Horse
    c) Dog d) Goat

26. The mortality rate of tetanus is higher in the following species
    a) Sheep and goat b) Horse
    c) Pigs d) Young ruminants

27. Ascending tetanus is common in the following
    a) Dog and cat b) Sheep and goat
    c) Horse d) All the above

28. Descending tetanus is common in the following
    a) Horse b) Dog and cat
    c) Sheep and goat d) All the above

29. The recommended dose of antitoxins for sheep and goat
    a) 200-300 I.U b) 1000-5000 I.U
    c) 10,000-20,000 I.U d) None of the above

30 Transmission of anthrax may occur by
    a) Direct contact with infected animal
    b) Ingestion of undercooked meat
    c) Mechanical carriage of spores by arthropods
    d) All the above

31. A complete necropsy of the animals is contraindicated in the following disease
    a) Brucellosis b) Anthrax
    c) Listeriosis d) Black leg

32. Inflammation of the mammary gland is not the characteristic feature in one of the following pathogens
    a) *Staphylococcus aureus* b) *Escherichia coli*
    c) *Leptospira interrogans* d) *S. agalactiae*

33. Limber neck is a clinical feature in sheep caused by
    a) *Clostridium botulinum* b) *Clostridium septicum*
    c) *Clostridium perfringens* d) *Clostridium novyi*

34. Casoni's test is used in the diagnosis of

a) Echinococcosis
b) Flukes
c) Anthrax
d) None of the above

35. The most common method of transmission of anthrax in cattle is

a) Ingestion
b) Inhalation
c) Percutaneous
d) Both a and b

36. Pica in cattle predisposes the following disease

a) Rinderpest
b) Anthrax
c) Salmonellosis
d) Foot and Mouth disease

37. The following is an effective sporicide when applied on soil during anthrax outbreaks

a) 3% Peracetic acid
b) 2% Phenol
c) 2% Formalin
d) None of the above

38. The effective method of eradication of tuberculosis in cattle is

a) Test and slaughter
b) Vaccination
c) Elimination of carriers
d) All the above

39. Increased shedding of *M. paratuberculosis* in faeces may occur due to the increased intake of

a) Dietry calcium
b) Dietry iron
c) Dietry protein
d) Both a and b

40. Most outbreaks of botulism in cattle are caused by the following neurotoxins of *Cl. botulinum*

a) Type A
b) Type B
c) Type C
d) Both a and b

41. Which organ is majorly involved in anthrax?

a) Kidney
b) Spleen
c) Liver
d) Heart

42. Involvement of lymph nodes is a characteristic feature in the following diseases except

a) Epizootic lymphangitis
b) Glanders
c) Ulcerative lymphangitis
d) All the above

43. Ingestion of preformed toxin is the main method of transmission of the following disease

    a) Tetanus
    b) Enterotoxaemia
    c) Braxy
    d) Botulism

44. Concurrent infection with following pathogens predisposes liver damage in bacillary haemoglobinuria except

    a) *Fusobacterium necrophorum*
    b) *Fasciola hepatica*
    c) *Cysticercus tenuicollis*
    d) *Pasteurella multocida*

45. Which one of the following is the most common and frequent route of transmission of Salmonella in farm animals?

    a) Faecal-oral route
    b) Nasal route
    c) Wound contamination
    d) Conjunctival route

46. Copper coloured liver is the characteristic pathological finding in

    a) Fowl typhoid
    b) Fowl cholera
    c) Pullorum disease
    d) All the above

47. Chronic form of glanders characterized by

    a) Pulmonary form
    b) Skin form
    c) Nasal form
    d) All the above

48. Strauss test is used in the diagnosis of following diseases except

    a) Brucellosis
    b) Strangles
    c) Actinobacillosis
    d) Glanders

49. Joint-ill is characterized by

    a) Omphalitis
    b) Omphalophlebitis
    c) Urachitis
    d) All the above

50. Passive transfer of maternally derived antibodies depends on

    a) Formation of colostrum with high concentration of immunoglobulin in the dam
    b) Ingestion of adequate quantity of colostrum by the neonates
    c) Efficient absorption of colostral immunoglobulins by the newborns
    d) All the above

51. Improperly fermented silage may be a risk factor for the following disease

a) Nervous coccidiosis
b) Toxico infectious botulism
c) Listeriosis
d) Hepatoencephalopathy

52. Enteric salmonellosis usually occurs in calves of the age

a) Birth to 2 weeks
b) 2-6 weeks
c) 6-10 weeks
d) 10-15 weeks

53. Thick-walled abscesses on the soft tissues of tongue and cervical lymph nodes are most commonly associated with

a) Actinomycosis
b) Tuberculosis
c) Actinobacillosis
d) Caseous lymphadenitis

54. Which one of the following pathogen is not involved in the etiology of joint-ill?

a) *Mycoplasma* sp.
b) *Erysipelathrix* sp.
c) *Corynebacterium* sp.
d) *Mycobacterium* sp.

55. Joint-ill is a disease of foals, affects mostly at the age group of

a) 1 week
b) 2 weeks
c) 1 month
d) Less than 6 months

56. Diphtheritic pox is seen in the following disease

a) Cow pox
c) Fowl pox
b) Horse pox
d) Contagious pustular stomatitis

57. The route of infection for joint-ill in lambs is

a) Oral route
b) Umbilicus
c) Reproductive tract
d) All the above

58. A group of baby chicks showing trouble in breathing, opened mouth, extended necks and gasping for air can be suspected for

a) Mycoplasma infection
b) Streptococcus infection
c) Staphylococcous infection
d) Aspergillus infection

59. Salmonellosis should be differentially diagnosed from

a) Coccidiosis
b) Pasteurellosis
c) Colibacillosis
d) All the above

60. The route of infection in salmonellosis is
    a) Respiratory tract b) Alimentary tract
    c) Genital tract d) Both b and c

61. The route of infection for arthritis in calves is
    a) Reproductive tract b) Oral route
    c) Umbilicus d) All the above

62. Drug that is very effective in treating shipping fever with no withdrawal period is
    a) Penicillin b) Tilmycosin
    c) Oxytetracyclin d) Gentamycin

63. The route of infection for arthritis in foals is
    a) Reproductive tract b) Umbilicus
    c) Nasal route d) All of the above

64. Tetanus has to be differentiated from
    a) Rabies b) Milk fever
    c) Strychnine poisoning d) All the above

65. Enterotoxemia of lambs can be prevented by
    a) Addition of antibiotic to feed
    b) Proper nutritional management
    c) Feeding a high grain diet
    d) Addition of sulphas to water

66. False negative tuberculin results may occur in
    a) Advanced stage of tuberculosis
    b) Heavily parasitized cattle
    c) Recently calved cow
    d) All the above

67. Actinomycosis in pig is characterized by
    a) Tumour in mammary gland
    b) Bursitis
    c) Lumpy jaw
    d) None of the above

68. Screening of a cattle herd against brucellosis should be by
    a) 2-mercaptoethanol test
    b) Complement fixation test
    c) Rose-bengal plate test
    d) Milk ring test

69. Nervous form of Listeriosis is common in
    a) Cattle
    b) Sheep
    c) Pigs
    d) Both a and b

70. Joint-ill in neonates is characterized by
    a) Inflammation of joints or synovial membrane
    b) Allergic reaction in the joints
    c) Immune mediated reaction in the joints
    d) None of the above

71. Sprorotrichosis, a fungal disease mainly affects the following
    a) Horses
    b) Cattle
    c) Dogs
    d) Pigs

72. The fungus *Sporotrichous schenkii* in the tissue phase is
    a) Cigar shaped
    b) Lemon shaped
    c) Pyriform shaped
    d) Oval

73. The reservoirs of the sporotrichosis are
    a) Wood
    b) Water
    c) Cattle
    d) Deer

74. The drug recommended for the treatment of *S. schenckii* is
    a) Penicillin
    b) Itraconazole
    c) Co-trimazole
    d) Oxytetracycline

75. The primary lesion of *Coccidiodes immitis* is
    a) Gastritis
    b) Pulmonary
    c) Genital
    d) All the above

76. The host affected by coccidioidosis is
    a) Cattle
    b) Pig
    c) Poultry
    d) Dog

77. The breed which is resistant to anthrax is
    a) Algerian sheep
    b) Merino sheep
    c) Jamunapari goat
    d) All the above

78. Which one of the following is a dimorphic fungus?
   a) *Candida* b) *Cryptococcus*
   c) *Histoplasma* d) All the above

79. Which one of the following is called as pseudoglanders?
   a) Histoplasmaosis b) Cryptococcosis
   c) Ringworm d) Strangles

80. The dermatophyte which mainly affects cattle is
   a) *T. verrucosum* b) *T. mentagraphytes*
   c) *M. gypseum* d) All the above

81. OIE-FAO Reference Lab- for avian flu is located at the following countries
   a) Japan b) USA
   c) UK d) All the above

82. Periodic ophthalmia in horses is caused by
   a) Leptospirosis b) Babesiosis
   c) Glanders d) Theileriosis

83. Brain like corrugation in distal small intestine of cattle is seen in
   a) Tuberculosis b) Johne's disease
   c) Rinderpest d) Haemorrhagic septicaemia

84. Quarantine period for brucellosis is
   a) 7 days b) 15-30 days
   c) 60- 90 days d) 120-365 days

85. Death in tetanus is due to
   a) Anaemia b) Asphyxia
   c) Anoxia d) Anuria

86. Timber tongue refers to the bacterial disease
   a) Actinobacillosis b) Actinomycosis
   c) Tetanus d) Grass tetany

87. The case fatality rate in black leg is
   a) 25% b) 50%
   c) 75% d) 100%

88. Vaginal mucus agglutination test is used for the following disease
    a) Campylobacteriosis b) Trichomonosis
    c) Brucellosis d) All the above

89. The type of vaccine recommended during the outbreak of IBR is
    a) Intranasal b) Intraocular
    c) Intramuscular d) Subcutaneous

90. Which one of the following interferes with the clotting mechanism?
    a) Parvo virus b) Ephemeral fever virus
    c) FMD d) CD

91. In fowl pox, the inclusion bodies are called as
    a) Guarnier bodies b) Elementary bodies
    c) Negri bodies d) Bollinger bodies

92. Iatrogenic transmission is possible in the following disease
    a) Anaplasmosis b) Rabies
    c) FMD d) None of the above

93. Diseases that are not in existence, but may be introduced at any time in the population are referred to as
    a) Exotic b) Endemic
    c) Exzootic d) Enzootic

94. The OIE/FAO World Reference Laboratory for FMD is located at
    a) UK b) USA
    c) India d) Japan

95. The etiological agent of Malta fever was first isolated in 1887 by
    a) David Bruce b) Bang
    c) Louis Pasteur d) Robert Koch

96. Contagious mastitis in dairy animals can also be called as
    a) Subclinical mastitis b) Environmental mastitis
    c) Clinical mastitis d) Acute mastitis

97. Rarefying osteomyelitis caused by actinomycosis is seen in
    a) Shoulder bones b) Lumbar vertebrae
    c) Skull d) Mandible

98. All pathogenic leptospires are grouped into
    a) *Leptospira biflexa* b) *Leptospira interrogans*
    c) *L. Icterohaemorrhagiae* d) *L. Pomona*

99. The strain which is used in the preparation of modified parvo viral vaccine is
    a) Cornell strain b) Manhatten strain
    c) Onderstepoort d) CVS

100. Clutching of toes in poultry is a characteristic feature of the disease
    a) IBD b) ILT
    c) Marek's disease d) Avian leukosis

101. Inflammatory oedema of throat in haemorrhagic Septicaemia is characteristic sign in
    a) Pigs b) Cattle
    c) Horse d) Goats

102. Passive immunity in horses can be conferred by administration of
    a) Tetanus toxoids b) Tetanus antitoxins
    c) Hyperimmune serum d) All the above

103. Which one of the following is intracellular in nature?
    a) *Listeria monocytogenes* b) *Leptospira canicola*
    c) *Manheima haemolytica* d) *Burkholderia mallei*

104. Bovine viral diarrhea can cause depletion of
    a) Thrombocytes b) RBCs
    c) Leukocytes d) Neutrophils

105. In Rose Bengal Plate test, the sample used for screening is
    a) Blood b) Serum
    c) Faeces d) Aborted fetal fluid

106. Nephritis seen in leptospirosis is
    a) Pyaemic b) Interstitial
    c) Glomerular d) All the above

107. The prominent lesion observed cattle died of anthrax is
    a) Splenomegaly b) Hepatomegaly
    c) Nephritis d) Pericarditis

108. Mastitis caused by *Staphylococcus aureus* in ewes results in the condition called

a) Blue bag b) Clinical mastitis
c) Subclinical mastitis d) Contagious mastitis

109. Langhan type giant cells are seen in

a) Tuberculosis b) Rinderpest
c) Gumboro's disease d) Fowl pox

110. Rabies virus spreads from the brain via the following to reach the saliva

a) Facial nerve b) Glossopharyngeal nerve
c) Both a and b d) Olfactory nerve

111. A tubercle nodule is formed of

a) Fibrous tissue b) Connective tissue
c) Granulomatous tissue d) None of the above

112. Blue tongue virus affects

a) Haemopoitic tissue b) Vascular endothelium
c) Both a and b d) Nervous tissue

113. Percutaneous transmission of *Strongyloides westeri* favours the transmission of

a) *C. pseudotuberculosis* b) Alpha virus
c) Lenti virus d) *Clostridium chauvoi*

114. The reservoir of hog cholera virus is

a) *Metastrongylus apri* b) *D. viviparus*
c) Glomerular tubules d) Soil

115. Which one of the following is favorable for anthrax outbreak?

a) Alkaline soil b) Acidic soil
c) High temperature d) Low humidity

116. Equine infectious anaemia is transmitted by

a) *Stomoxys spp* b) *Culicoides spp*
c) *Ixodes spp* d) Both b and c

117. The host which is resistant to Johne's disease is
   a) Pig b) Buffaloe
   c) Cattle d) Goat

118. The recommended method for eradication of FMD in enzootic areas is
   a) Vaccination b) Test and slaughter
   c) Quarantine d) Culling

119. Which one of the following is an effective disinfectant for anthrax spores?
   a) 3% Per acetic acid b) 2% Sodium hydroxide
   c) 4% Sodium carbonate d) All the above

120. The risk factor responsible for enterotoxaemia is
   a) Heavy grain feeding b) Low lying area
   c) Exotic breed d) All the above

121. The most common method of transmission of anthrax in cattle is
   a) Ingestion b) Inhalation
   c) Percutaneous d) Both a and b

122. Copper coloured liver is the characteristic pathological finding in
   a) Fowl typhoid b) Fowl cholera
   c) Pullorum disease d) All the above

123. Which one of the following disease is called swine plague?
   a) Hog cholera b) Transmissible gastro enteritis
   c) Atropic rhinitis d) Swine influenza

124. Which one of the following disease is called cattle plague?
   a) Apthous fever b) Rinderpest
   c) Ephemeral fever d) IBR

125. Which one of the following disease is called ox typhoid?
   a) Rinderpest b) Ephemeral fever
   c) FMD d) Malignant catarrhal fever

126. Which one of the following disease is called equine typhoid?
   a) Strangles b) African horse sickness
   c) Equine infectious anaemia d) Vesicular stomatitis

127. Which one of the following disease is called canine typhus?
  a) Canine distemper
  b) Infectious canine hepatitis
  c) Rabies
  d) Leptospirosis

128. Which one of the following diseases is referred to as fast moving disease?
  a) Infectious bovine rhinotracheitis
  b) Rift valley fever
  c) Malignant catarrhal fever
  d) FMD

129. Which one of the following disease is called canine influenza?
  a) Corona viral disease
  b) Canine distemper
  c) CPV-2 infection
  d) CPV-1 infection

130. Milk drop syndrome refers to
  a) Rota viral disease
  b) Coccidiosis
  c) Leptospirosis
  d) Haemorrhagic septicaemia

131. Flabby udder mastitis refers to the following disease
  a) Candidiasis
  b) Cryptococcosis
  c) Leptospirosis
  d) Aspergillosis

132. Limber neck is a characteristic sign in the following disease
  a) Botulism
  b) Tetanus
  c) Black disease
  d) None of the above

133. The symptoms of black quarters may resemble the signs of
  a) Anthrax
  b) Malignant oedema
  c) Acute lead poisoning
  d) All the above

134. Nagler's reaction is commonly employed in the diagnosis of
  a) *Clostridium novy* type A
  b) *Clostridium septicum*
  c) *Clostridium perfringens*
  d) *Clostridium haemolyticum*

135. In BVD, mucosal disease explodes in the persistently infected cattle when subsequent infection occurs with
  a) Cytopathic BVDV
  b) Non-cytopathic BVDV
  c) Virulent strain
  d) Pathogenic strain

136. Ephemeral fever causes the inflammation of

a) Joints
b) Muscles
c) Lymph nodes
d) All the above

137. Bacillary haemoglobinuria in ruminants is predisposed by infestation of the metacestode

a) *Cysticercus tenuicollis*
b) *Cysticercus cerebralis*
c) *Cysticercus ovis*
d) None of the above

138. Mallein test is recommended in the diagnosis of

a) Strangles
b) Glanders
c) Equine infectious anaemia
d) Equine rhinoracheitis-1

139. The most commonly encountered pathogenic *Salmonella* in all species is

a) *S. Paratyphi*
b) *S. Entertidis*
c) *S. Typhi*
d) *S. Typhimurium*

140. In miliary tuberculosis, development of nodules occurs in

a) Lungs
b) Kidney
c) Bones
d) All the above

141. Viral pneumonia in calves maybe complicated by the bacteria

a) *Salmonella*
b) *Mycoplasma*
c) *E.coli*
d) All the above

142. In swine fever, the major mechanism of virus perpetuation in epizootics caused by low virulent strains is

a) Latent infection
b) Persistent infection
c) Reservoir status
d) Amplification of virus

143. Pruritus is characteristic of Pseudorabies in the following host

a) Horse
b) Cow
c) Dog
d) Pig

144. The OIE recommended screening test for brucellosis is

a) Tube agglutination test
b) c-ELISA
c) I- ELISA
d) Rose Bengal plate test

145. Clinical form of Johne's disease occurs only at the age of

a) >2-3 years b) 1 year
c) 6 months d) >5 years

146. The pathogen commonly involved in environmental mastitis is

a) *E. coli* b) *Mycoplasma*
c) *Staphylococcus aureus* d) *Streptococus agalactiae*

147. Contagious mastitis is referred to as

a) Summer mastitis b) Subclinical mastitis
c) Environmental mastitis d) Fungal mastitis

148. Environmental mastitis is referred to as

a) Clinical mastitis b) Cold mastitis
c) Bacterial mastitis d) Fungal mastitis

149. Emphyema of guttural pouche in horses is a complication of

a) Strangles
b) Glanders
c) Equine herpes virus infection
d) Histoplasmosis

150. Vegetative endocarditis and non-suppurative arthritis are seen in pigs suffering from

a) Chronic erysipelas b) Acute erysipelas
c) Per acute erysipelas d) Sub acute erysipelas

151. The most important necropsy finding in anthrax is

a) Splenomegaly b) Oozing of clotted blood
c) Haemorrhagic enteritis d) All the above

152. The neurotoxic clostridia pathogenic to sheep are

a) *Clostridium perfringens* b) *Clostridium chauvoi*
c) *Clostridium novy* type A d) *Clostridium welchii*

153. Edema disease in pigs is caused by

a) Salmonella b) *E. coli*
c) Rota virus d) Corona virus

154. Marker vaccines are generally practiced with the objective of
   a) Differentiation of herpes viral diseases
   b) Eradication of herpes viral infections from the herd
   c) To differentiate the infected and vaccinated individuals
   d) All the above

155. Most of the FMD outbreaks in India are due to
   a) Serotype O
   b) Serotype A
   c) Serotype C
   d) Serotype Asia 1

156. The characteristic clinical sign of African horse sickness is oedema in
   a) Eyelids
   b) Joints
   c) Muscles
   c) None of the above

157. Rinderpest was declared globally eradicated in the year
   a) 2010
   b) 2011
   c) 2012
   d) 2013

158. Rinderpest infection was eradicated in India in the year
   a) 1994
   b) 2005
   c) 2000
   d) 2002

159. The Pan Asiatic serotype of foot and mouth disease vims
   a) Serotype Asia 1
   b) Serotype C
   c) Serotype A
   d) Serotype O

160. The following serotype of FMD is rare in India
   a) Serotype A
   b) Serotype C
   c) Serotype O
   d) Serotype Asia 1

161. The signs of FMD in cattle are very similar to
   a) Rinderpest
   b) Theileriosis
   c) IBR
   d) Ephemeral fever

162. Encephalitic form of listeriosis is characteristic in
   a) Pigs
   b) Horses
   c) Cattle
   d) Dogs

163. The characteristic sign of vesicular exanthema in pigs is
   a) Blotching of ears
   b) Diamond lesions
   c) Ouchy gait
   d) Suppurative arthritis

164. The cow side test for the diagnosis of mastitis is
   a) White side test
   b) California mastitis test
   c) Chloride test
   d) Strip cup test

165. Atropic rhinitis in pigs is caused by
   a) *P. multocida* type A
   b) *P. haemolytica* type A
   c) *Pasteurella multocida* type B
   d) *P. multocida* type D

166. Botulism in cattle is caused commonly
   a) By the ingestion of spores of *C. botulinum*
   b) By the ingestion of toxins of *C. botulinum*
   c) By the ingestion of bacilli of *C. botulinum*
   d) By the inhalation of toxins of *C. botulinum*

167. The maintenance host for *Leptospira icterohaemorrhagiae* is
   a) Dog
   b) Pigs
   c) Rodents
   d) Lagomorphs

168. African swine fever is commonly transmitted by
   a) Mosquitoes
   b) Biting flies
   c) Ticks
   d) Physical contact

169. The strain commonly used for vaccination against *Brucella abortus* in cattle is
   a) Sterne
   b) S19
   c) Weybridge
   d) Cotton strain

170. The vaccine strain which can be used in eradication of brucellosis is
   a) S19
   b) S 45/20
   c) Rev -1
   d) RB51

171. Strangles is characterized by
   a) Nodules in the upper respiratory tract.
   b) Inflammation of upper respiratory tract
   c) Inflammation of lower respiratory tract
   d) Nodules in lower respiratory tract

172. The disinfectant which is effective in the control of FMD is

a) 2% Sodium carbonate
b) 1% Sodium hydroxide
c) 4% Sodium carbonate
d) 1% formalin

173. The reservoir involved in the transmission of FMD is

a) Wild-beast
b) Deer
c) Elephants
d) Rodents

174. Clinical and acute viral pneumonia in calves is caused by

a) PI-3
b) BRSV
c) Rhino virus
d) Adeno virus

175. In cattle, abortion due to brucellosis occurs in pregnancy in its

a) 1st trimester
b) 2st trimester
c) 3st trimester
d) Any stage

176. Anton's test is used in the diagnosis of

a) Louping -ill
b) Listeriosis
c) Rabies
d) Tuberculosis

177. Which one of the following is true?

a) *Bacillus anthracis* is a gram positive, motile and non-capsulated bacterium.
b) *Bacillus anthracis* is a gram positive, non-motile and capsulated bacterium.
c) *Bacillus anthracis* is a gram positive, motile and capsulated bacterium.
d) *Bacillus anthracis* is a spore forming, motile and non-capsulated bacterium.

178. Vesicular stomatitis is a disease which primarily affects

a) Pigs
b) Horses
c) Cattle
d) Dogs

179. One dose of anthrax vaccine contains

a) 1 million spores of *B.anthracis*
b) 2 million spores of *B.anthracis*
c) 5 million spores of *B.anthracis*
d) 10 million spores of *B.anthracis*

180. Air borne spread of foot and mouth disease virus can occur over land

a) Not beyond 8 km b) Not beyond 10 km
c) Not beyond 30 km d) Not beyond 60 km

181. Which one of the following is true in case of ephemeral fever?

a) It causes drastic drop in milk production
b) It causes severe dehydration and emaciation
c) It causes enteritis and keratoconjunctivitis
d) None of the above

182. Immunotolerance due to BVD in cattle occurs as a result of the

a) Recognition of the virus as "non-self" by the host
b) Entry of the virus during first 240 days of pregnancy
c) Recognition of the virus as "self" by the host
d) None of the above

183. Double haemolysis in blood agar is a diagnostic finding of

a) *C. perfringens* b) *Brucella suis*
c) *B. anthracis* d) *P. haemolytica*

184. Farcy refer to the

a) Thickening of blood vessels in limb
b) Thickening of lymph vessels in limb
c) Lymphadenitis in face and surrounding tissues
d) Cutaneous ulcers in the limb area

185. Tetanus anti toxins can confer immunity for a period of

a) 1 week b) 2-3 weeks
c) 1 month d) 2-3 months

186. FMD causes high fatality in the following group

a) Calves b) Suckling calves
c) Pregnant cows d) Exotic adults

187. Which one of the following is the common method of transmission in FMD?

a) Inhalation b) Ingestion
c) Cutaneous d) Venereal

188. Which one of the following is a common feature in FMD?

a) Abortion
b) Encephalitis
c) Stomatitis
d) Mastitis

189. Which one of the following is not a sequel to FMD?

a) Hypertrichosis
b) Panting
c) Enteritis
d) Mastitis

190. Which one of the following is the primary method of transmission in swine fever?

a) Inhalation
b) Ingestion
c) Transplacental
d) Louse

191. Persistent infection in pigs is an important feature in

a) Swine fever
b) Erysipelas
c) Salmonellosis
d) Pasteurellosis

192. Exposure to the following disease causes high mortality in pigs with swine fever

a) Pasteurellosis
b) Salmonellosis
c) Erysipelas
d) Both a and b

193. Pseudorabies is highly fatal in

a) Sheep and goats
b) Cattle
c) Pigs
d) Both a and b

194. In pseudorabies, respiratory disorders are mainly observed in

a) Piglets
b) Fatteners and weaners
c) Sows
d) Boars

195. Marker vaccines of pseudorabies has the following advantage

a) Serological differentiation of infected and vaccinated pigs
b) Long lasting protection
c) Avoids shedding of virus and its spread within herd
d) All of the above

196. Pseudorabies in pigs causes the following signs

a) Central nervous system signs

b) Respiratory signs
c) Reproduction disorders
d) All of the above

197. Louping-ill in sheep is predisposed by the following diseases

a) Ehrlichiosis b) Clostridial diseases
c) Listeriosis d) Acute lead poisoning

198. The following organ is affected in sheep with louping-ill

a) Liver b) Intestine
c) Brain d) Uterus

199. Leaping-ill in sheep is characterized by

a) Encephalitis b) Meningitis
c) Bouncing gait d) All the above

200. The following disease should be differentiated from louping-ill in sheep

a) Ehrlichiosis b) Moneziasis
c) Anaplasmosis d) Scrapie

201. Reduced efficacy of vaccines in equine influenza is due to

a) Antigenic drift b) Vectors spread
c) Seasonal change d) Virulence of virus

202. Equine influenza should be differentiated from the following diseases

a) Corona viral infection b) Rhino viral infection
c) Parvo viral infection d) Rota viral infection

203. The following is the method of transmission in equine distemper

a) Ingestion b) Tick bite
c) Inhalation d) Fly bite

204. The following is the vector most commonly involved in the transmission of African horse sickness

a) Tabanus b) Stomoxys
c) *Culex spp* d) *Culicoides spp*

205. African horse sickness is caused by the following agent
    a) Alpha virus
    b) Retrovirus
    c) *Malleomyces mallei*
    d) None of the above

206. Which one of the following is not an arthropod borne disease?
    a) Equine infectious anemia
    b) African horse sickness
    c) EEE
    d) None of the above

207. Which one of the following is a mosquito-borne disease?
    a) Equine infectious anemia
    b) Equine encephalitis
    c) African horse sickness
    d) None of the above

208. Coggin'ss test is employed in the diagnosis of the following disease
    a) Equine infectious anemia
    b) African horse sickness
    c) Glanders
    d) Strangles

209. Which one of the following should be differentiated from equine infectious anemia?
    a) Strangles
    b) African horse sickness
    c) Strongylosis
    d) Glanders

210. The transmission cycle of Eastern equine encephalitis occurs between
    a) Birds & mosquitoes
    b) Mosquitoes & horses
    c) Mosquitoes and humans
    d) Birds and horses

211. The amplifying hosts in the transmission of Eastern and Western equine encephalitis are
    a) Mosquitoes
    b) Horses
    c) Birds
    d) Pigs

212. Canine distemper in dogs results in catarrhal enteritis due to the secondary infection with
    a) Morbilli virus
    b) *E.coli*
    c) *Salmonella* spp.
    d) *Bordotella*

213. Old dog encephalitis is common in infection with following agent
    a) Parvo virus
    b) Herpes virus
    c) Adeno virus
    d) Morbilli virus

214. The following is not the clinical sign of canine distemper in dogs
a) Chorea
b) Chewing gum type seizure
c) Blindness
d) None of the above

215. Cutaneous form of canine distemper results in vesiculo pustular pattern in
a) Abdomen
b) Inner thigh
c) Both a and b
d) Head

216. The laboratory animal of choice for canine distemper is
a) Ferret
b) Mouse
c) Guinea pig
d) Rabbit

217. Age of first vaccination against canine distemper is
a) 6 weeks
b) 12 weeks
c) 3 months
d) 6 months

218. The source of infection in the transmission of infectious canine hepatitis is
a) Urine
b) Blood
c) CSF
d) Saliva

219. Which one of the following is not a clinical feature in infectious canine hepatitis?
a) Glaucoma
b) Enteritis
c) Tucked up abdomen
d) Bronchopneumonia

220. Canine papillomatosis causes muco-cutaneous tumors in
a) Perineum
b) Mouth
c) Abdomen
d) All the above

221. "Fading pups" is a Symptom in puppies caused by
a) Canine minute virus (CMnV)
b) Canine Parvo virus (CPV-2)
c) Corona virus
d) Morbilli virus

222. Which of the following is common in puppies of less than 10 weeks old infected with parvovirus?
a) Respiratory
b) Nervous form
c) Cardiac form
d) Intestinal form

223. Which one of the following is not true for swine vesicular exanthema?
   a) The disease is caused by calci virus
   b) Abortion occurs in infected pregnant pigs
   c) Vesicles occur in snout, abdomen, teat and foot
   d) The disease is non-zoonotic

224. Vesicular exanthema is a disease of
   a) Cattle   b) Pigs
   c) Cattle and pigs   d) Goats

225. Which one of the following is not antigenically related to rinderpest virus?
   a) Canine distemper   b) Measles
   c) PPR   d) Vesicular stomatitis

226. The following method is important in the transmission of rinderpest
   a) Ingestion   b) Inhalation
   c) Vector bite   d) All the above

227. The host which is relatively resistant to rinderpest is
   a) Cattle   b) Buffaloe
   c) Pig   d) Goat

228. The following laboratory test can differentiate rinderpest from PPR
   a) AGID   b) CIEP
   c) c-DNA probe   d) Neutralization test

229. The animal employed for inoculation test in the diagnosis of rinderpest is
   a) Cattle   b) Guinea pig
   c) Mouse   d) Hamster

230. The primary method of transmission of vesicular stomatitis in cattle is
   a) Ingestion   b) Inhalation
   c) Vector borne   d) All the above

231. Which one of the following disease causes high mortality in young calves?
   a) Foot and mouth disease   b) Vesicular stomatitis
   c) Malignant catarrhal fever   d) Both a and b

232. Which one of the following is not true for the disease vesicular stomatitis in cattle?
   a) It causes high mortality in young calves
   b) Clinically indistinguishable from FMD
   c) Vesicle may be absent frequently in the oral mucosa.
   d) Rarely causes vesicles on feet and udder

233. Development of runts in the pregnant cattle is a feature in the following disease
   a) Malignant catarrhal fever
   b) Foot and mouth disease
   c) Rinderpest
   d) Mucosal disease

234. For declaration of a country freedom from rinderpest, the country should not have reported the disease for
   a) 2 years b) 3 years
   c) 5 years d) 10 years

235. Carrier sow syndrome occurs in swine infected with
   a) Calicivirus b) Flavi virus
   c) Asfi virus d) Pesti virus

236. Pseudorabies causes nervous disorders primarily in
   a) Sows and Boars b) Fatteners
   c) Adult pigs d) Piglets

237. Which one of the following is a non-arthropod borne disease?
   a) Equine infectious anaemia b) Sleeping sickness
   c) Equine influenza d) Peste- equina

238. The OIE recommended test for detection of rabies is
   a) FAT b) RFFIT
   c) RREID d) Mouse neutralization test

239. Ranikhet disease is caused by
   a) Adeno virus type I b) Birna virus
   c) Herpes virus d) Rubula virus

240. Parvovirus is readily inactivated by

i) 2% Formalin
ii) Chloroform
iii) 2% Sodium hydroxide

a) i
b) ii and iii
c) i and iii
d) i, ii and iii

241. Single dose of rabies vaccine should contain the antigenic titre of

a) ≥ 1.5 IU
b) 1.5 IU to 2.0 IU
c) 2.0 IU to 2.5 IU
d) 2.5 IU to 5.0 IU

242. 'Pearl eye' in birds is caused by

a) Corona virus
b) Paramyxovirus
c) Herpes virus
d) Adeno virus

243. Mortality in fowl pox is higher when lesions occur in

a) Comb and wattle
b) Feet and vent
c) Mouth and esophagus
d) Eyes

244. Which one of the following is not of public health significance?

a) Cow pox
b) Buffalo pox
c) Fowl pox
d) Pseudos cow pox

245. The inclusion bodies of fowl pox virus seen in the epithelial cells are

a) Bollinger bodies
b) Borrel granules
c) Guarnier bodies
d) None of the above

246. Major loss in IB is due to

a) Decreased egg production
b) Poor quality eggs
c) Heavy mortality
d) All the above

247. Catarrhal tracheitis, bronchitis and caseous plugs in the lower trachea and bronchi are the indications of

a) IB
b) ILT
c) Avian influenza
d) ND

248. In cattle infected with MCF, the characteristic lesions are seen in

a) Head and eye form
b) Alimentary form
c) Reproductive form
d) Nervous form

249. The following clinical sign is not a feature of MCF
 a) Nervous sign b) Keratoconjunctivitis
 c) Respiratory sign d) Infertility

250. Latency of infection is not a feature in the following
 a) IBR b) MCF
 c) BVD d) All the above

251. Coital exanthema in cattle is caused by
 a) IBR b) Rinderpest
 c) FMD d) None of the above

252. Which one of the following is not a common feature in IBR
 a) Pink muzzle b) Infertility
 c) Enteritis d) Broncho pneumonia

253. The recommended method of diagnosis for scrapie is
 a) Histopathology b) ELISA
 c) Culture and Isolation d) None of the above

254. The recommended measure for eradication of scrapie is
 a) Slaughter of infected animals
 b) Destruction of familial lines of infected sheep
 c) Improvement of genetically susceptible breeds
 d) All the above

255. Which one of the following pathogen is not commonly involved in the viral pneumonia of calves?
 a) PI-3 b) BRSV
 c) Mycoplasma d) Rhino virus

256. Fatal pneumonia in calves is caused by
 a) BRSV b) Mycoplasma
 c) PI-3 d) All the above

257. Antigenic mutation is a phenomenon caused by the following agent
 a) Oncorna virus b) Flavi virus
 c) Pesti virus d) Paramyxo virus

258. The early finding of bovine lymphomatosis in cattle is
   a) Bloat b) CHF
   c) Oedema d) Lymph node enlargement

259. Ability of the virus to reach the CNS depends upon
   a) Distance of the bite b) Virulence of strain of virus
   c) Concentration of the virus d) All the above

260. Avian dermatophytosis is caused by
   a) *Trichophyton megninii* b) *Coccidioides immitis*
   c) *Histoplasma capsulatum* d) None of the above

261. Which one of the following is a superficial fungal disease?
   a) Favus b) Histoplasmosis
   c) Coccidioidomycoses d) All the above

262. Which one of the following is an immunosuppressive disease?
   a) ND b) IB
   c) IBD d) Avian encephalomyelitis

263. The source of infection for the fungal disease sporotrichosis is
   a) Birds b) Plant material
   c) Horse d) Cat

264. Which one of the following is similar to sporotrichosis?
   a) Ulcerative lymphangitis b) Glanders
   c) Histoplasmosis d) All the above

265. Wood's light method is used in the diagnosis of
   a) *Microsporon canis* b) *M. gypseum*
   c) *T. equi* d) All the above

266. FMD causes high mortality in the following
   a) Heifers b) Exotic cattle
   c) Buffalo d) Cross bred cattle

267. Ingestion is the primary method of transmission of FMD in the following
   a) Cattle b) Sheep
   c) Pigs d) All the above

268. The primary complication of FMD in cattle is
a) Mastitis
b) Enteritis
c) Panting
d) None of the above

269. *Haematopinus suis* can transmit the following
a) Hog cholera
b) Vesicular exanthema
c) FMD
d) All

270. Persistent infection due to BVD occurs in cattle at the following gestation period
a) <30 days
b) <60 days
c) <120 days
d) >60 days

271. Pruritus is rare in the following species
a) Cattle
b) Sheep
c) Pigs
d) All the above

272. Louping ill is predisposed by
a) *Ehrlichia spp*
b) *Babesia*
c) *Anaplasma spp*
d) All the above

273. The reservoirs of equine encephalitis virus are
a) Swamp birds
b) Pigeons
c) Pigs
d) Mosquitoes

274. The respiratory infection in canine distemper is complicated by
a) *Bordotella*
b) Parainfluenza
c) Rhino virus
d) Adeno virus

275. The age of first vaccination for canine rabies is
a) 2 months
b) 6 months
c) 3 months
d) 4-5 months

276. Which one of the following vaccine for rabies is contraindicated?
a) Nervous tissue
b) Diploid cell
c) Vero cell
d) All the above

277. The important source of infection for vesicular exanthema in swine is
a) Nasal droplet
b) Swills
c) Water
d) Semen

278. Non cytopathic virus of swine fever in sow results in
a) Thin sow syndrome
b) Carrier sow syndrome
c) Runts
d) Enteritis

279. The characteristic lesion in Marek's disease is
a) Pink eye
b) Pearl eye
c) Blue eye
d) Glaucoma

280. The elementary bodies in fowlpox infection is called as
a) Borrel bodies
b) Bollinger bodies
c) Inclusion bodies
d) Guarnier bodies

281. The primary method of transmission of sheep pox is
a) Ingestion
b) Fly bite
c) Inhalation
d) Venereal

282. Systemic infection is common in the following
a) Swinepox
b) Sheeppox
c) Horsepox
d) Buffalopox

283. Mechanical transmission of swine pox by louse is important in the following
a) Cattle
b) Sheep
c) Pigs
d) All the above

284. The kind of vaccine used in the eradication of IBR is
a) Inactivated vaccine
b) Virulent vaccine
c) Attenuated vaccine
d) Marker vaccine

285. The primary source of infection in Rubarth's disease is
a) Blood
b) Urine
c) Saliva
d) Semen

286. An effective, cheap and easily available chemical that can be used as disinfectant against FMD virus is
a) Na_2Co_3
b) NaoH
c) Formalin
d) KOH

287. Erosions on the tip of cheek papillae especially at the commissures of the mouth is characteristic lesions in
a) Contagious ecthyma
b) Sheep pox
c) Goat pox
d) Lumpy skin disease

288. Most commonly used highly sensitive, specific laboratory test for the immunodiagnosis of rabies is

a) ELISA
b) FAT
c) REID
d) RFFIT

289. African horse sickness is transmitted biologically by

a) *Aedes sp.*
b) *Culicoides sp.*
c) *Ixodes sp.*
d) All the above

290. Accumulation of prion protein in the neuronal tissue is responsible for the non-febrile fatal disease of the sheep called

a) Spongiform encephalopathy
b) BSE
c) Scrapie
d) MSE

291. Enlargement of liver is characteristic lesion in adult chicken which die due to

a) Newcastle disease
b) Gumboro's disease
c) Avian leukosis
d) Inclusion body hepatitis

292. Epidemic tremor refers to

a) Infectious avian encephalomyelitis
b) Thiamine deficiency
c) Hypoglycaemia
d) Marek's disease

293. The method of transmission of ringworm in domestic animals is

a) Physical contact
b) Aerosol
c) Inhalation
d) All the above

294. Lymphoid lesions are observed in the following disease of poultry

a) Marek's disease
b) Avian leukosis
c) IBD
d) Fowl pox

295. Turkey egg kidney is a characteristic postmortem lesion in swine of

a) Corona viral disease
b) Calici viral disease
c) Pestiviral disease
d) Picorna viral disease

296. Rabies in animals is caused by

a) Lyssa virus genotype 1 b) Lyssa virus genotype 2
c) Lyssa virus genotype 36 d) Rhabdo virus

297. The mortality percentage in infectious bursal disease of poultry varies between

a) 10-20 percent b) 5-10 percent
c) 80-100 percent d) 50-80 percent

298. 'Turkish towel" appearance of mucosa of crop in poultry is a characteristic finding of the following

a) Candidiasis b) Histoplasmosis
c) Dermatophytosis d) Aflatoxicosis

299. The following strain of Ranikhet disease is more virulent

a) Lentogenic b) Mesogenic
c) Velogenic d) All the above

300. Tick borne encephalitis group comprises the following

a) Louping-ill b) Scrapie
c) Borreliosis d) Ehrlichiosis

301. Contagious ecthyma is a viral disease of

a) Sheep b) Goat
c) Cow d) All the above

302. Acute undifferentiated diarrhoea of newborn farm animals is the synonym for

a) Colibacillosis b) Salmonellosis
c) Rota viral diarrhoea d) All the above

303. Modified Parvo viral strain used in Parvocine vaccine is

a) Onderstepoort b) C-1309
c) Manhatten d) Cornell

304. The viral strain used in BHK-21 rabies vaccine is

a) Wister b) Cornell
c) Pitman Moore d) CVS

305. A thin thready pulse with week, rapid heart sounds is of diagnostic value in

a) Canine distemper b) Kennel cough
c) Infectious canine hepatitis d) Parvoviral enteritis

306. IBR virus is antigenically related to

a) Equine rhinopneumonitis b) Pseudorabies
c) Bovine mammilitis d) Malignant catarrhal fever

307. BHV 1.2 infection in cattle causes

a) Genital disease b) Respiratory disease
c) Nervous disease d) All the above

308. *Dictyocaulus viviparous* infection in cattle activates the latent infection of the disease

a) Ascariasis b) IBR
c) Parainfluenza d) Mycoplasmosis

309. The site of latency of infectious bovine rhinotracheitis virus is

a) Lymph nodes b) Trigeminal nerve
c) Respiratory tract d) All the above

310. Abortion by IBR virus is caused in the following trimester of pregnancy

a) First b) Second
c) Third d) All the above

311. The calf with congenital abnormalities when infected with Ncp virus of BVD is called

a) PI calf b) Carrier
c) Runt d) Latent calf

312. Aphthous fever is caused by

a) Aphtha virus b) Picorna virus
c) Enterovirus d) Vesiculo virus

313. FMD is characterized by the formation of vesicles in

a) Foot and oral cavity b) Foot, mouth and udder
c) Teats and mouth d) All the above

314. Most of the FMD outbreaks in India are due to the following serotypes

a) O, Asia-1 and A
b) O, A and C
c) O and Asia
d) O and Asia-1

315. In FMD, the amplifier hosts are

a) Pigs
b) Elephants
c) Buffaloes
d) Wild ruminants

316. FMD causes death in young calves due to lesion in

a) GI tract
b) Heart
c) Pituitary gland
d) All the above

317. Pig plague is a contagious disease caused by

a) Calici virus
b) Pesti virus
c) Picorna virus
d) Orthomyxo virus

318. The virus of hog cholera is antigenically closely related to

a) Swine dysentery virus
b) TGE virus
c) BVD virus
d) IBR virus

319. The intermediate host and reservoir for hog cholera virus is

a) Earth worm
b) Beetles
c) Slugs
d) Lung worm

320. In swine fever, the major mechanism of virus perpetuation in epizootics caused by low virulent strains is

a) Latent infection
b) Subclinical infection
c) Reservoir status
d) Persistent infection

321. The important method of transmission of African swine fever is

a) Tick bite
b) Mosquitoe bite
c) Ingestion
d) Fly bite

322. The life cycle involved in the transmission of African swine fever is

a) Culex- birds
b) Tick-warthog
c) Aedes- warthog
d) All the above

323. Pseudorabies in piglets causes disorders of

a) Genital system
b) Muscular system
c) Nervous system
d) Respiratory system

324. In pseudorabies, cattle act as
   a) Maintenance host b) Primary host
   c) Aberrant host d) Dead end host

325. The common sign in cattle affected with pseudorabies is
   a) Pruritus b) Diarrhoea
   c) Salivation d) Abortion

326. Pseudorabies, a disease of pigs is caused by the virus
   a) SHV-1 b) SHV-2
   c) Rhadino virus d) Alpha herpes viridae

327. Louping-ill is a disease of primarily
   a) Goats b) Calves
   c) Lambs d) All the above

328. Trembling-ill in sheep is characterized by
   a) Bouncing gait b) Circling
   c) Twitching d) None of the above

329. The transmitting agent of louping –ill is
   a) Ixodes ricinus b) Stomoxys sp
   c) Rhiphicephalus sp d) All the above

330. Russian spring encephalitis is transmitted by the method
   a) Ingestion b) Tick bite
   c) Both ingestion and tick bite d) None of the above

331. Equine typhoid fever is caused by
   a) Influenza virus b) Alpha herpes virus
   c) Retro virus d) *Streptococcus equi*

332. Equine influenza in foals causes severe and fatal
   a) Bronchopneumonia b) Anaemia
   c) Bronchitis d) Dyspnoea

333. Equine distemper refers to
   a) Histoplasmosis b) African horse sickness
   c) Equine encephalitis d) Equine influenza

334. African horse sickness virus is antigenically related to the virus of

a) Border disease
b) Mucosal disease
c) Equine encephalitis
d) Bluetongue

335. The vector involved in the biological transmission of African horse sickness is

a) Mosquitoes
b) *Ixodes* sp
c) *Stomoxys* sp
d) *Culicoides* sp

336. Coggin's disease is caused by

a) Retro virus
b) Orthomyxo virus
c) Flavi virus
d) Orbi virus

337. Equine infectious anemia is transmitted by the biting insects, commonly

a) *Tabanus* sp
b) Stable fly
c) Both a and b
d) *Chrysobs* sp

338. Virus of equine infectious anemia is antigenically related to the virus of

a) Feline immunodeficiency
b) Human immunodeficiency
c) Avian leukosis
d) Bovine leukemia

339. The important source of infection in the transmission of swamp fever in horses is

a) Nasal discharge
b) Saliva
c) Faeces
d) Blood

340. Equine infectious anemia virus causes damage to

a) RBC
b) RES cells
c) RBC and RES cells
d) RBC and epithelial cells

341. The clinical sign of Coggin's disease is

a) Haemorrhage in the visceral organs
b) Edema of the orbital fossa and eyelids
c) Haemorrhage in the mucosae
d) Frothy and bloody nasal discharge

342. Coggins test is employed in the diagnosis of
   a) Equine infectious anaemia b) Equine arteritis
   c) Equine encephalitis d) Equine rhinopneumonitis

343. The international trade test recommended for screening swamp fever is
   a) Coggin's test b) Strauss test
   c) CAMP test d) ELISA

344. The pathogenic effect of tick borne fever in sheep is
   a) Immunosuppression b) Secondary infection
   c) Septicaemia d) All the above

345. Lymphnode involvement is common in the following equine infection
   a) *H. capsulatum* b) *Burkholderia mallei*
   c) *Sporotrichous schenckii* d) All the above

346. Air sacculitis is characteristic of the following infection
   a) *M. gallisepticum* b) Coronal virus
   c) *S. Pullorum* d) *P. multocida*

347. Agglutination test is commonly used in the diagnosis of
   a) Bacillary white diarrhoea b) Chronic respiratory disease
   c) Campylobacteriosis d) All the above

348. Which one of the following is contagious?
   a) Candidiasis b) Aspergillosis
   c) Canine histoplasmosis d) Dermatophilosis

349. Tram-track appearance is a characteristic colonial morphology of
   a) *D. congolensis* b) *M. haemolytica*
   c) *C. pseudotuberculosis* d) *L. monocytogenes*

350. Acute and fatal anaplasmosis can occur in the following
   a) Calves b) Suckling calves
   c) Lambs d) Adult Cattle

351. Iatrogenic transmission is a method of transmission in
   a) Anaplasmosis b) Candidiasis
   c) Tetanus d) All the above

352. Which one of the following is commonly susceptible to candidiasis?
   a) Cattle b) Chicken
   c) Turkey d) All the above

353. The complication of tick borne fever is commonly due to
   a) Staphylococcal pyaemia b) Brucellosis
   c) Listeriosis d) Pasteurellosis

354. Formation of chlamydospores in the corn meal agar is characteristic of the following
   a) Apergillosis b) Histoplasmosis
   c) Sporotrichosis d) Candidiasis

355. Which one of the following is not a feature of aspergillosis in cattle?
   a) Abortion
   b) Mastitis
   c) Granulomatous pneumonia
   d) Enteritis

356. Which one of the following is a Category- A bioterrorism agent?
   a) *B. anthracis* b) *C. botulinum* toxin
   c) *Yersinia pestis* d) All the above

357. The disease which is transmitted by cat scratch is
   a) *Sporotrichus schenckii* b) *Bartonella henslae*
   c) *P. multocida* type A & C d) All the above

358. The reservoirs of *Coccidioides immitis* are
   a) Pigeons b) Rabbits
   c) Rodents d) Water birds

359. The complication of tick borne fever in sheep is due to
   a) Immunosuppression b) Listeriosis
   c) Abortion d) All the above

360. Inflammation of lymphoid tissue is common in the following equine infection
   a) *H. capsulatum* & *B. mallei* b) *Leptospira* & *S. equi*
   c) *C. pyogenes* d) All the above

361. Omphalitis in chicken is characteristic of the following infection

a) *E. coli* b) *M. synoviae*
c) *S. Pullorum* d) *M. gallisepticum*

362. Which one of the following is an opportunistic disease?

a) Candidiasis b) Mycoplasmosis
c) Aflatoxicosis d) Q fever

363. Pallisade appearance is a characteristic colonial morphology of

a) *D. congolensis* b) *M. haemolytica*
c) *C. pseudotuberculosis* d) *L. monocytogenes*

364. 'Thrush' is a fungal lesion observed in

a) Poultry b) Cattle
c) Sheep d) All the above

365. Pasture fever is caused by

a) *A. phagocytophilum* b) *A. marginale*
c) *A. ovis* d) None of the above

366. Formation of germ tubes in serum agar is characteristic of

a) Candidiasis b) Histoplasmosis
c) Sporotrichosis d) Apergillosis

367. The reservoir of *histoplasma capsulatum* is

a) Pigeons & bats b) Rabbits & wild ruminants
c) Rodents & pigeons d) Water birds

368. Which one of the following is the sporucidal agent for anthrax?

a) 3% per acetic acid b) 2% Sodium bicarbonate
c) 2% Cresol d) 2% Phenol

369. Gram's staining is not useful in the diagnosis of

a) *Leptospira* & *Brachyspira* b) *B. burgdorferi*
c) *B. anserina* d) All the above

370. The lethal and necrotizing toxin causing classical enterotoxaemia is

a) Epsilon b) Enterotoxin
c) Iota d) Alpha

371. Descending tetanus is common in the following
    a) Man
    b) Cat
    c) Dog
    d) All the above

372. Spastic paralysis which occurs in tetanus is due to
    a) Inhibition of GABA
    b) Inhibition of Ach
    c) Inhibition of Ach and glycine
    d) None of the above

373. Strauss's test is used in the diagnosis of following diseases except
    a) Strangles
    b) Brucellosis
    c) Actinobacillosis
    d) Glanders

374. RB-51 vaccination can be recommended for the following
    a) Adults
    b) Pregnant cows
    c) Bulls
    d) All the above

375. Which one of the following results in clinical mastitis?
    a) *Mycoplasma*
    b) *Staph. aureus*
    c) *Streptococcus agalactiae*
    d) *E.coli*

376. Vegetative endocarditis and non-suppurative arthritis are seen in pigs suffering from
    a) Sub acute erysipelas
    b) Acute erysipelas
    c) Per acute erysipelas
    d) Chronic erysipelas

377. Latency is characteristic in the following disease
    a) Strangles
    b) Anthrax
    c) Glanders
    d) Salmonellosis

378. Agglutination test is commonly used in the diagnosis of
    a) Pullorum disease
    b) Brucellosis
    c) Campylobacteriosis
    d) All the above

379. The following is highly susceptible to anaplasmosis
    a) Exotic cattle
    b) Adult cattle
    c) Well nourished cattle
    d) All the above

380. Iatrogenic transmission is common in
   a) Anaplasmosis b) Aspergillosis
   c) Tetanus d) All the above

381. Which one of the following is saprophytic ?
   a) *Aspergillus sp* b) *Histoplasma*
   c) *Sporotrichous sp* d) All the above

382. Which one of the following is a Category- A bioterrorism agent?
   a) *B. anthracis* b) *C. botulinum* toxin
   c) *Yersinia pestis* d) All the above

383. The stain which is useful in diagnosis of fungal dseases is
   a) Lactophenol cotton blue
   b) Periodic acid Schiff
   c) Gomori's methanamine silver stain
   d) All the above

384. Allergic test can be employed in the diagnosis of
   a) Tuberculosis b) Brucellosis
   c) Johne's disease d) All the above

385. The immunodominant site for leptospires is
   a) Renal tubules b) Aquous humour of eye
   c) Mammary gland d) All the above

386. The risk factor for the increased incidence of Johne's disease is
   a) Parturition b) Acidity of the soil
   c) Overcrowding d) All the above

387. The source of infection for listeriosis is
   a) Faeces b) Chicken meat
   c) Milk d) All the above

388. The case-fatality is generally high in
   a) Brucellosis b) Black quarters
   c) Tuberculosis d) None of the above

389. The laboratory animal of choice for pasteurellosis is
   a) Guinea pig b) Rabbit
   c) Mice d) None of the above

390. Incubation temperature for the fungal culture is
   a) 37°C in blood agar
   b) 25°C in Sabaoraud's agar
   c) 37°C in Sabaoraud's agar
   d) 25°C in blood agar

391. Which one of the following is not dimorphic?
   a) *Histoplasma capsulatum*
   b) *Candida albicans*
   c) *Sporotrichus schenckii*
   d) *Coccidioides immitis*

392. The diagnostic form of *Histoplasma sp* that can be identified in tissues is
   a) Hyphae
   b) Yeast cells
   c) Macroconidia
   d) Microconidia

393. Facial edema is a sign of the following disease
   a) *M. synoviae*
   b) *M. gallisepticum*
   c) *E. coli*
   d) None of the above

394. Vertical transmission is not a feature in the following infection
   a) *Mycoplasma gallisepticum*
   b) *E. coli*
   c) Salmonella Pullorum
   d) S. Gallinarum

395. Facial eczema, a mycotoxicosis is commonly observed in
   a) Cattle
   b) Sheep
   c) Goat
   d) All the above

396. The immunosuppression caused by aflatoxicosis in animals is due to
   a) Leucopenia
   b) Inhibition of protein synthesis
   c) Neutropenia
   d) All the above

397. Coggin's test is based on the principle of
   a) AGID
   b) ELISA
   c) Animal inoculation
   d) None of the above

398. Marbling of lungs in cattle is characteristic in the disease caused by
   a) *Mycoplasma mycoides* subsp *mycoides* SC
   b) *Mycoplasma mycoides* subsp.*mycoides* LC
   c) *Mycoplasma capricolum* subsp. *capripneumonia*
   d) *Mycoplasma capricolum* subsp. *capricolum*

399. Botulism, a saprozonoses commonly occurs in animals due to
   a) Ingestion of *C. botulinum* toxins in the feed
   b) Ingestion of *C. botulinum* spores in the feed
   c) Entry of *Cl. botulinum* toxins through wound
   d) Inhalation of *Cl. botulinum* spores in soil

400. Pullorum disease and fowl typhoid can be differentiated by
   a) Culture
   b) Carbohydrate reaction
   c) Copper coloured lesions
   d) Agglutination test

401. The characteristic finding of *M. gallinarum* infection in turkeys is
   a) Swelling of infra orbital sinus
   b) Swelling of frontal sinus
   c) Swelling of joints
   d) Respiratory rales

402. The bacteria which is 'ribbon' like under Gram's staining is
   a) *Campylobacter* sp.
   b) *Actinomyces* sp.
   c) *Erysipelothrix* sp.
   d) *Microsporon canis*

403. The pathognomonic lesion in canine Lyme disease is
   a) Encephalitis
   b) Arthritis
   c) Icterus
   d) Nephritis

404. Bronze liver is a characteristic lesion in the diagnosis of
   a) *S.* Dublin
   b) *S.* Gallinarum
   c) *S.* Abortus equi
   d) *S.* Typhimurium

405. The common method of transmission for Q fever is
   a) Inhalation
   b) Ingestion
   c) Cutaneous
   d) None of the above

406. The following is called as hog cholera bacillus
   a) *S.* Abortus equi
   b) *S.* Abortus ovis
   c) *S.* Cholerae suis
   d) *S.* Enteritidis

407. The bacteria which causes typhlocolitis in growing pigs is
   a) *Brachyspira hyodysentriae*
   b) *Salmonella* Cholerae suis
   c) *Erysipelothrix* sp.
   d) *E. coli*

408. In dermatophilosis of sheep, skin lesions lead to the characteristic appearance of

a) Paint brush b) Nodular lesions
c) Pallisade d) Vesicular lesions

409. Chinese letter appearance is characteristic of the following

a) *Actinobacillus sp.* b) *Campylobacter sp.*
c) *Actinomyces sp.* d) *Corynebacterium sp.*

410. The reservoirs of equine encephalitis are

a) Horses b) Pigs
c) Birds d) Pigeons

411. The hosts involved in the transmission cycle of eastern equine encephalitis are

a) Birds and mosquitoes b) Mosquitoes and horses
c) Bats and horses d) Pigeons and horses

412. Canine distemper in dogs is characterized by

a) Encephalitic form b) Ocular form
c) Respiratory form d) All the above

413. Ray fungus like appearance is characteristic of the following

a) *Campylobacter sp.* b) *Dermatophilus sp.*
c) *Actinomyces sp.* d) *Corynebacterium sp.*

414. The dead end hosts of equine encephalitis are

a) Horses b) Pigs
c) Cattle d) Birds

415. The foremost sign seen in canine distemper is

a) Nervous sign b) Pustules
c) Respiratory sign d) Enteric sign

416. Fatal infection with canine distemper virus results in the depletion of

a) Lymphocytes b) Red blood cells
c) Thrombocytes d) Nerve cells

417. Canine distemper virus in dogs has the tropism for

a) Epithelial tissue
b) Lymphoid tissue
c) Nervous tissue
d) All the above

418. Canine distemper in dogs results in exudative pneumonia due to the infection with the commensal

a) *Bordetella bronchiseptica*
b) Rhino virus
c) Canine adeno virus-1
d) Parainfluenza virus

419. The hosts involved in the transmission cycle of Venezualen equine encephalitis are

a) Birds and horses
b) Mosquitoes and horses
c) Bats and horses
d) Rodents and mosquitoes

420. Infectious canine hepatitis causes blue eye due to

a) Corneal edema and iridocyclitis
b) Corneal ulcers
c) Glaucoma
d) Blepharospasm

421. Papilloma virus in dogs causes

a) Oral form
b) Ocular form
c) Cutaneous form
d) All the above

422. Increased replication of parvo virus in young puppies is favoured by the concurrent parasitism by

a) *Ancylostomum sp.*
b) *D. latum*
c) *Babesia canis*
d) *Dipylidium caninum*

423. Complete protection against canine parvo viral infection is conferred by

a) T lymphocytes
b) B lymphocytes
c) IgA
d) IgG

424. The common forms of clinical signs in canine parvovoiral infection are

a) Intestinal & cardiac form
b) Intestinal & respiratory form
c) Encepahalitic & Intestinal form
d) Intestinal & ocular form

425. The most common virus which causes enteritis in dogs is
   a) Calici virus b) Parvo virus
   c) Adeno virus d) Toga virus

426. Swine vesicular exanthema should be differentiated from
   a) Foot and mouth disease b) Swine vesicular disease
   c) Rinderpest d) All the above

427. GREP is developed for the eradication of rinderpest from the whole world by the year
   a) 2000 b) 2010
   c) 2015 d) 2005

428. Rinderpest was eradicated globally by the year
   a) 2010 b) 2011
   c) 2012 d) 2013

429. The list A disease of cattle which causes immune suppression is
   a) Rinderpest b) Foot and mouth disease
   c) IBR d) Catarrhal fever

430. Which one of the following is not a phase of rinderpest in cattle
   a) Erosive mucosal phase b) Diarrhoeic phase
   c) Convalescent phase d) Pulmonary phase

431. Rinderpest in goat can be differentiated clinically from PPR by the absence of the
   a) Enteritis b) Laminitis
   c) Stomatitis d) Pneumonia

432. The method of eradication of Rinderpest recommended by OIE is
   a) Culling b) Treatment
   c) Disinfection d) Slaughter

433. Vesicular stomatitis in cattle and pigs is indistinguishable from
   a) Rinderpest b) Foot and mouth disease
   c) Swine fever d) All the above

434. The amplifier hosts of vesicular stomatitis are
   a) Deer b) Horses
   c) Cattle d) Pigs

435. BVD virus is closely related to the virus of the disease
   a) Hog cholera
   b) Border disease of sheep
   c) Both a) and b)
   d) African swine fever

436. Mucosal disease develops when cattle persistently infected with non-cytopathic virus becomes super infected with
   a) Avirulent BVD virus
   b) BVD virus
   c) Cytopathic virus
   d) Pesti virus

437. A sudden epidemic disease of cattle causing fever, stiffness and lameness with recovery after 3 days is
   a) Malignant catarrhal fever
   b) Vesicular stomatitis
   c) Ephemeral fever
   d) Foot and mouth disease

438. Ephemeral fever in cattle is transmitted mainly by the bite of
   a) Stable fly
   b) Sand fly
   c) Deer fly
   d) Tse-tse fly

439. Strawberry lymph node is a characteristic necropsy finding of the viral disease
   a) Blue tongue
   b) Swine fever
   c) Peste-des petits ruminants
   d) Bovine viral diarrhoea

440. Non-cytopathic bovine viral diarrhoea virus in cattle results in
   a) Latent infection
   b) Persistent infection
   c) Subclinical infection
   d) Sterile immunity

441. Latent infection is the outcome of infection in cattle infected with
   a) Pesti virus
   b) Corona virus
   c) Morbilli virus
   d) Herpes virus

442. Ephemeral fever in cattle causes
   a) High morbidity and high mortality
   b) Low morbidity and low mortality
   c) Low morbidity and high mortality
   d) High morbidity and low mortality

443. Rinderpest in cattle results in the activation of latent infections since the virus causes

a) Thrombocytopenia b) Epitheliosis
c) Enteritis d) Immunosuppression

444. Keratoconjunctivitis in cattle is a characteristic sign of the disease

a) Malignant catarrhal fever b) IBR
c) Ephemeral fever d) Vesicular stomatits

445. In the control of infectious bovine rhinotracheitis, the vaccines which are advantageous over modified live virus vaccines are

a) Marker vaccines b) Intranasal vaccines
c) Tc vaccines d) Inactivated vaccines

446. The reservoir of classical swine fever virus is

a) Lung worm b) Earthworm
c) Pigs d) Wart hogs

447. Trembling-ill in sheep is transmitted by

a) *Ixodes ricinus* b) *Culicoides sp*
c) *I. dammini* d) *Tabanus sp*

448. The reservoir host of the virus causing equine encephalomyelitis is

a) Pigeons b) Poultry
c) Pigs d) Wild swamp birds

449. Potassium iodide is used in the treatment of

a) Anthrax b) Hamorrhagic septicaemia
c) Leptospirosis d) Actinomycosis

450. Leptospirosis is associated with

a) Renal dysfunction b) Hepatic dysfuntion
c) Meningitis d) All the above

451. Capsular stain used in the staining of *Bacillus anthracis* is

a) Loefflers methylene blue b) Polychrome methylene blue
c) Methylene blue d) Methyl violet

452. Peral's disease is the synonym of

a) Johne's disease b) Tuberculosis
c) Actinomycosis d) Histoplasmosis

453. Causative agent of timber tongue is
  a) *Actinomyces bovis* b) *Actinobacillus equili*
  c) *Actinobacillus lignieresi* d) *Coccidioidus immitis*

454. Greasy pig disease caused *Staphylococcus hyicus* is also known as
  a) Ulcerative cellulitis b) Exudative dermatitis
  c) Caseous lymphadenitis d) Infectious polyarthritis

455. Pulpy kidney disease is caused by *Closteridium perfringens*
  a) Type A b) Type C
  c) Type C d) Type D

456. Silage consumption is associated with
  a) Leptospirosis b) Salmonellosis
  c) Brucellosis d) Listeriosis

457. Stormont test is used in the diagnosis of
  a) Leptospirosis b) Salmonellosis
  c) Tuberculosis d) Johne's disease

458. The neurotoxin produced by *Clostridium tetani* is
  a) Tetanolysin b) Tetanospasmin
  c) Haemolysin d) None of the above

459. The etiological agent of the barbone disease is
  a) *Pasteurella multocida* b) *Clostridium septicum*
  c) *Bacillus anthracis* d) *Pasteurella haemolytica*

460. Shaker foal syndrome in horses is caused by
  a) *Clostridium botulinum* b) *Streptococcus equi*
  c) Alpha virus d) *Clostridium tetani*

461. Which one of the following is referred to as ray fungus?
  a) *Actinomyces bovis* b) *A. pleuropnemoniae*
  b) *Streptococcus equi* d) None of the above

462. Purpura haemorrhagica is a sequel of
  a) Strangles b) Glanders
  c) Pseudoglanders d) Histoplasmosis

463. Which one of the following is less susceptible to tetanus?
   a) Cattle b) Sheep
   c) Horses d) Dog

464. Which one of the following is resistant to tetanus?
   a) Cat b) Poultry
   c) Pig d) Dog

465. The serotype of *Pasteurella multocida* which causes haemorrhagic septicaemia in India is
   a) E b) B
   c) C d) D

466. Snuffles in rabbits is caused by *P. multocida*
   a) Type A b) Type C
   c) Type C d) Type D

467. Atropic rhinitis in pigs is caused by *P. multocida* type D and
   a) *Bordetella bronchiseptica* b) *Mannheimia haemolytica*
   c) *A. pleuropneumoniae* d) None of the above

468. Abortion causing zoonotic disease
   a) Leptospirosis b) Brucellosis
   c) Both a and b d) Pasteurellosis

469. The clinical signs in cardiac form of African horse sickness is
   a) Oedema of head b) Limping
   c) Hyperaesthesia d) Paddling

470. Young calves are resistant to
   a) Pseudorabies b) FMD
   c) Vesicular stomatitis d) BVD

471. Sudden death is common in
   a) Enterotoxaemia b) Acute leptospirosis
   c) Struck d) All the above

472. The species susceptible to vesicular exanthema is
   a) Sheep and goat b) Cattle
   c) Dog d) Swine

473. The following diseases are transmitted by arthropods
   a) Bovine ephemeral fever   b) Anthrax
   c) Vesicular stomatitis   d) All

474. Important clinical signs of tetanus in horses are
   a) Trismus   b) Stiffness of lambs
   c) Opisthotonus   d) All

475. The continent which is free from rabies is
   a) Australia and Newzealand   b) Asia
   c) Africa   d) None

476. "Chewing gum" type of seizure is characteristic of the following disease
   a) Canine distemper   b) Infectious hepatitis
   c) Parvo viral enteritis   d) Rabies

477. In the transmission of African horse sickness, dog act as
   a) Silent host   b) Biological carrier
   c) Reservoir host   d) Mechanical carrier

478. Malignant form of sheep pox is common in
   a) Adults   b) Lambs
   c) Ewes   d) Rams

479. Day old chicks are vaccinated against the following disease
   a) IBD   b) ILT
   c) MD   d) IB

480. The complement fixation test used in the diagnosis of avian leucosis is
   a) Cason's test   b) Ascoli's test
   c) Straus test   d) Cofal test

481. The biotype of virus which causes persistent infection in foetus is
   a) Non-cytopathic virus   b) Cytopathic virus
   c) Classical BVD virus   d) Non-classical BVD virus

482. Rabies is an example for
   a) Convalescent carrier   b) Incubatory carrier
   c) Latent carrier   d) All the above

483. Rabies viral protein detected by fluorescent antibody test is
a) Glycoprotein b) Nucleoprotein
c) Matrix protein d) None of the above

484. 'Katta' is the synonym of
a) PPR b) Rinderpest
c) Foot and Mouth disease d) Blue tongue

485. Causative agent of blue tongue is
a) Orbi virus b) Aptha virus
c) Picorna virus d) Herpes virus

486. HVT vaccine is used against
a) Marek's disease b) Infectious laryngotracheitis
c) Infectious bronchitis d) Avian leucosis

487. Red nose is also called as
a) BVD b) IBR
c) MCF d) Vesicular stomatits

488. Sore nose is caused by
a) Vesi virus b) Vesiculo virus
c) Rhadino virus d) Varicella virus

489. Milker's nodules develop in the hands of milkers after milking goats suffering from
a) FMD b) Mastitis
c) Pseudocow pox d) None of the above

490. Foot and mouth disease in pigs should be differentiated from
a) Vesicular exanthema b) Vesicular stomatitis
c) Swine vesicular disease d) All the above

491. Rinderpest in cattle should be differentiated from
a) BVD b) Vesicular stomatitis
c) FMD d) All the above

492. The wild animals playing important role in the spread of rabies in India are
a) Monkey b) Fox
c) Jackel d) All the above

493. In India, 97% cases are due to

a) Dog bite | b) Cat bite
c) Dog and cat bite | d) All the above

494. IBD is also called as

a) Gumboro disease | b) Pearls eye
c) Fowl plague | d) None of the above

495. Marek's disease vaccine is given at the age of

a) Day 0 | b) Day 7
b) Day 14 | d) Day 21

496. For diagnosis of rabies, the choice of laboratory animal is

a) Suckling mice | b) Guinea pig
c) Rabbit | d) None of the above

497. The choice of laboratory animal for foot and mouth disease is

a) Mice | b) Guinea pig
c) Hamster | d) None of the above

498. The control of equine infectious anemia is considered difficult due to

a) Persistent infection | b) Inapparent form
c) Subclinical infection | d) None of the above

499. The most fatal form of African horse sickness is

a) Cardiac form | b) Pneumonic form
c) Intestinal form | d) None of the above

500. Dwarfing and curling of embryo are the characteristic changes observed in ECE inoculated with the isolates of

a) IB | b) IBD
c) ND | d) Avian flu

501. The important source of infection for Marek's disease is

a) Faeces | b) Bursa of fabricious
c) Feather follicle | d) Liver tissue

502. The level of protective neutralizing antibody titre in serum of anti-rabies vaccinated individual is

a) $\geq$ 0.5 IU per ml | b) $\geq$ 1.0 IU per ml
c) $\geq$ 2.0 IU per ml | d) $\geq$ 2.5 IU per ml

503. Wet and dry forms are the clinical forms of the following disease

a) Sheep pox b) Swine pox
c) Equine pox d) Fowl pox

504. The virus which results in CRD in association with Mycoplasma is

a) Herpes virus b) Corona virus
c) Retro virus d) None of the above

505. Laying watery white egg by chicken is associated with the disease

a) ILT b) Avian encephalitis
c) Fowl pest d) Infectious bronchitis

506. Malignant catarrhal fever causes fatal disease in

a) Sheep b) Goat
c) Rabbits d) Cattle

507. Inapparent or subclinical malignant catarrhal fever occurs in

a) Sheep b) Pig
c) Deer d) Cattle

508. In cattle infected with MCF, the signs characteristic are

a) Respiratory b) Encephalitic
c) Ocular d) None of the above

509. Which one the following is the risk factor for malignant catarrhal fever?

a) Housing of cattle and sheep together
b) Vector population in the infected area
c) Movement of carrier cattle
d) Movement of pigs in the susceptible population

510. The respiratory disease in cattle of viral origin is

a) MCF b) BRSV
c) IBR d) PI3

511. Infectious bovine rhinotracheitis is considered important in dairy cattle since the economic losses are due to

a) Abortion b) Infertility
c) Mortality in calves d) All the above

512. Transmissible spongiform encephalopathy in sheep is clinically characterized by
   a) Ascending paralysis b) Tremors
   c) Gait abnormalities d) Circling

513. Mouth thrush refers to the disease caused by
   a) Respiratory syncytial virus b) Vesiculo virus
   c) Rhadino virus d) PI3 virus

514. 'Sore mouth' refers to the disease caused by
   a) Aphtha virus b) Vesiculo virus
   c) Morbilli virus d) BHV-1

515. Snot sickness in cattle is caused by the virus
   a) Rhadino virus b) Varicella virus
   c) Para influenza-3 virus d) Herpes virus

516. When compared to conventional viruses, prion does not posses
   a) DNA b) RNA
   c) Both a and b d) Nucleocapsid

517. The secondary pathogens primarily involved in the shipping fever complex are
   a) *Mycoplasma* sp b) *Pasteurella* sp
   c) *Haemophilus* sp d) All the above

518. The highly fatal disease of cattle which causes malignant neoplasia of reticuloendothelial system is
   a) Bovine leucosis b) Rindepest
   c) Meliodosis d) BSE

519. IBR is highly fatal in the following
   a) Buffaloe b) Cattle
   c) Calves d) Lambs

520. Which one of the following is the reservoir of malignant catarrhal fever?
   a) Deer b) Rabbit
   c) African buffaloes d) Elephants

521. Which one of the following is a clinical form of bovine leucosis?
   a) Classical form
   b) Enzootic form
   c) Persistent form
   d) All the above

522. The indicator host for foot and mouth disease is
   a) Sheep
   b) Pig
   c) Cattle
   d) Goat

523. In the malignant form of FMD, the signs are
   a) Cardiac
   b) Enteric
   c) Abortion
   d) All the above

524. Pan Asiatic serotype of FMD is
   a) O
   b) A
   c) Asia -1
   d) C

525. The number of strains in FMD virus is more than
   a) 10
   b) 100
   c) 1000
   d) 80

526. The antigenic part which is highly immunogenic in FMDV is
   a) VP1
   b) VP2
   c) VP3
   d) VP4

527. FMD infected cattle can act as reservoir for a period of
   a) 1 year
   b) 2 years
   c) 3 years
   d) 4-5 years

528. The carrier status in FMD is due to the latency of the virus in
   a) Oesophago- pharynx
   b) Nasal cavity
   c) Renal tubules
   d) Tonsils

529. Which one of the following is the most important risk factor in the spread of foot and mouth disease?
   a) Movement of cattle
   b) Lack of vaccination
   c) Multiple serotypes
   d) None of the above

530. In India, rabies cases occur due to the dog bite which accounts for
   a) 90 per cent
   b) 97 per cent
   c) 50 per cent
   d) 95 per cent

531. ABC is a programme employed in the control of rabies in

a) Dog b) Cattle
c) Human d) All the above

532. Coccidiodomycosis is a disease of

a) Cattle b) Horse
c) Dog d) All the above

533. Coccidiodomycosis is characterized by the following signs

a) Respiratory b) Ocular
c) Digestive d) None of the above

534. The method recommended in the elimination of prions from carcass is

a) Disinfection with 5% phenol
b) Incineration
c) Gamma Irradiation
d) None of the above

535. The amplifier host in equine encephalitis is

a) Horse b) Pig
c) Dog d) Birds

536. The dead end host for leptospirosis is

a) Birds b) Man
c) Cattle d) Rodents

537. The reservoir for African horse sickness is

a) Dog b) Elephant
c) Both a and b d) Donkeys

538. Secondary infection in cattle affected with cow pox may result in

a) Abortion b) Pyaemia
c) Enteritis d) Mastitis

539. The primary method of transmission of cowpox is

a) Physical contact b) Inhalation
c) Ingestion d) Vector bite

540. The primary method of transmission of sheep pox is

a) Physical contact b) Inhalation
c) Ingestion d) Vector bite

541. In India, 2 per cent of the rabies cases reported are due to the bite by

a) Dog b) Cat
c) Fox d) Bat

542. The most common form of African horse sickness is

a) Cardiac form b) Pulmonary form
c) Mixed form d) None of the above

543. The serotypes of African horse sickness virus prevalent worldwide are

a) 9 b) 24
c) 4 d) 19

544. The type of vaccine commercially available for African horse sickness is

a) Killed b) Live attenuated
c) Toxoids d) Genetically engineered

545. The host involved in the transmission cycle of Venezualen equine encephalitis is

a) Rodents b) Birds
c) Horse d) Pigs

546. The susceptible host involved in the transmission cycle of EEE and WEE is

a) Rodent b) Bird
c) Horse d) Pig

547. Favus, a disease of birds causes lesions in

a) Comb b) Wattle
c) Both a and b d) Intestine

548. Triple E in horses is caused by

a) Alpha virus b) Orbi virus
c) Retro virus d) Orthomyxo virus

549. White comb disease in birds is caused by the fungus

a) *Microsporon canis* b) *T. verrucosum*
c) *T. mentagraphytes* d) *Trichophyton gallinae*

550. Honey comb like appearance is caused by dermatophytes in

a) Chicken b) Cattle
c) Horse d) Pigs

551. Asbestos like lesions are characteristic in

a) Dog b) Poultry
c) Cattle d) Pigs

552. Which one of the following equine disease is highly fatal?

a) WEE b) African horse sickness
c) Equine infectious anaemia d) Equine influenza

553. Woods lamp is used in the diagnosis of

a) *Microsporon canis* b) *T. verrucosum*
c) *T. mentagraphytes* d) *Trichophyton megnini*

554. The drug of choice for histoplasmosis in dogs is

a) Amphotericin B b) Miconazole
c) Griseofulvin d) Tetracycline

555. *Histoplasma capsulatum* in horses causes the disease

a) Epizootic lymphangitis b) Ulcerative cellulitis
c) Lymphadenitis d) Lymphadenitis

556. Which one of the following is the OIE list A disease of equines?

a) EEE b) African horse sickness
c) Equine infectious anaemia d) Equine influenza

557. Sleeping sickness in horses is caused by

a) *Streptococcus equi* b) Orbi virus
c) *Pseudomonas mallei* d) Alpha virus

558. Histoplasmosis in animals is characterized by the granulamatous lesions in

a) Respiratory tract b) Digestive tract
c) Both a and b d) Brain

559. Mouth thrush in cattle refers to
   a) FMD
   b) Swine fevor
   c) Vesicular stomatitis
   d) Rinderpest

560. The most common host affected by histoplasmosis is
   a) Cattle
   b) Horse
   c) Pig
   d) Dog

561. The reservoirs of histoplasmosis are
   a) Pigs
   b) Horse
   c) Pigeons
   d) Dog

562. BRSV infection in cattle is clinically characterized by
   a) Broncho intertitial pneumonia
   b) Fibrinous pneumonia
   c) Bronchitis
   d) Rhinitis

563. Sporotrichosis is characterized by development of nodules on
   a) Skin
   b) Lungs
   c) Bronchi
   d) Kidney

564. The superficial fungal infection of the cornified epidermis and hair fibres is
   a) Dermatophilosis
   b) Sporotrichosis
   c) Histoplasmosis
   d) Dermatophytosis

565. Snotting sickness refers to
   a) Infectious bovine rhinotracheitis
   b) Pneumonic pasteurellosis
   c) Rhino virus
   d) Malignant catarrhal fever

566. The fungi involved in tinea are
   a) *Microsporon*
   b) *Trichophyton*
   c) *Epidermophyton*
   d) All the above

567. The dermatophytes causing ring worm in cattle are
   a) *Microsporon canis*
   b) *Trichophyton mentagrophytes*
   c) *T. verrucosum*
   d) All the above

568. The medium used for the growth of dermatophytes is
a) Sabouraud's dextrose agar b) Blood agar
c) Nutrient agar d) Meat broth

569. The reservoir for sporotrichosis is
a) Pigeons b) Horses
c) Decaying plants d) All the above

570. Mad dog syndrome refers to
a) Rabies b) Pseudorabies
c) Canine distemper d) None of the above

571. Mad cow disease refers to
a) Rabies b) Aujeszky's disease
c) BSE d) None of the above

572. Coital exanthema in cows and bulls is caused by
a) BHV-1.2 b) BHV-1.1
c) BHV -1.3 d) None of the above

573. Pink muzzle refers to the following disease
a) Classical malignant catarrh b) IBR
c) Para influenza -3 d) None of the above

574. The virus responsible for the respiratory disease of cattle is
a) Rhadino virus b) Varicella virus
c) Gamma herpes virinae d) None of the above

575. The site of latency for the alpha herpes virus is
a) Trigeminal nerve b) Lymphoid cells
c) RES cells d) Optic nerve

576. The site of latency for the gamma herpes virus is
a) Trigeminal nerve b) Lymphoid cells
c) RES cells d) Optic nerve

577. Marker vaccines are generally employed in the eradication of
a) IBR b) Pseudorabies
c) Both a and b d) Malignant catarrhal fever

578. Currently used marker vaccines in the control of IBR are
   a) Live attenuated b) Killed
   c) Toxoid d) DNA vaccines

579. The deletion protein in the commercial IBR vaccine is
   a) VP1 b) gE
   c) Tk gene d) gX

580. DIVA vaccines are employed in the field for
   a) Differentiation of infected and vaccinated animals
   b) Surveillance programme for a disease
   c) Eradication of a disease
   d) All the above

581. The period of immunity conferred by intranasal vaccines for IBR is
   a) 1 day b) 2 days
   c) 7 days d) 14 days

582. The disadvantage of modified live vaccines in the control of IBR is
   a) They are abortigenic in pregnant animals
   b) They may result in transmission of virus
   c) They may cause disease in young calves
   d) All the above

583. The advantage of intranasal vaccination for IBR is
   a) They stimulate more gamma interferons
   b) They stimulate more local antibodies
   c) They are not abortigenic in pregnant animals
   d) All the above

584. Temperature-sensitive (Ts) vaccines against IBR are administered by the following route
   a) Intranasal b) Intramuscular
   c) Intraocular d) Subcutaneous

585. IBR causes 100% mortality in the following
   a) Young Calves b) Yearlings
   c) Cows d) None of the above

586. The reservoir for infectious bovine rhinotracheitis is
a) Rodents b) Wild ruminants
c) Rabbit d) Birds

587. The difficulty in the eradication of IBR is due to
a) The latent infection in the infected animals
b) Reactivation of the infection in the recovered animals
c) Secondary bacterial infection in the infected animals
d) All the above

588. Blue eye syndrome is one of the complications of the following
a) Infectious canine hepatitis b) Canine distemper
c) Parvoviral enteritis d) Kennel cough

589. Haemorrhage in the thigh muscles of chickens is the lesion found in
a) Gumboro disease b) Marek's disease
c) Ranikhet disease d) Chicken infectious anaemia

590. Iatrogenic transmission is one of the modes of transmission in
a) Bovine leukosis b) Equine infectious anaemia
c) Tetanus d) All the above

591. Development of cutaneous nodules and ulcers on the limbs of horses is the clinical sign in
a) Histoplasmosis b) Glanders
c) Both a and b d) Strangles

592. Scrapie is a disease of small ruminants with high susceptibility to the breed
a) Merino b) Suffolk
c) Tellichery d) Jamnapari

593. Virus induced papillomas are seen in
a) Cattle b) Dog
c) Buffaloe d) All the above

594. Louping ill is transmitted by the tick
a) *Ixodes ricinus* b) *Ixodes persulcatus*
c) *Ixodes dammini* d) *Rhiphicephalus sanguneus*

595. *Salmonella* Pullorum from *S. Gallinarum* can be differentiated by

a) Culture b) Agglutination test
c) ELISA d) Biotyping

596. Horse pox is called as Jenner's pox when lesions are seen in

a) Head b) Leg
c) Trunk d) Face

597. Chronic form of anthrax is observed in

a) Pig b) Elephant
c) Sheep d) Goat

598. Pharyngitis in anthrax is a common sign in the following

a) Pig b) Cattle
c) Sheep d) Deer

599. BHV 1.2 virus in cattle causes

a) Neurological disease b) Respiratory disease
c) Genital disease d) Stomatitis

600. 'Mad-itch' refers to

a) Pseudorabies b) Rabies
c) BSE d) TSE

601. Conjunctivitis in cattle is a clinical feature due to the infection by

a) BHV-1 b) OHV-2
c) Both d) None of the above

602. Latent infection is the outcome of infection by

a) Pesti virus b) Calici virus
c) Retro virus d) Herpes virus

603. The secondary bacterial complication in BHV-1 infection is mainly due to

a) *Haemophilus* b) *Mycoplasma*
c) PI-3 d) *Pasteurella*

604. Which one of the following is a feature in IBR?

a) Rhinitis b) Tracheitis
c) Conjunctivitis d) All the above

605. The OIE recommended test for diagnosis of IBR virus is
   a) Agent identification in semen
   b) AGID
   c) FAT
   d) ELISA

606. The OIE recommended test for diagnosis of latent infection by IBR is
   a) ELISA b) PCR
   c) AGID d) FAT

607. Intracytoplasmic inclusion bodies can be seen in lesions of
   a) Swine Pox b) Influenza
   c) Rubarth's disease d) Marek's disease

608. Intranuclear inclusion bodies can be seen in
   a) ICH b) Rabies
   c) Marek's disease d) All the above

609. The international trade test for diagnosis of rabies in animals is
   a) Enzyme linked immunosorbent assay (ELISA)
   b) Flourescent antibody test (FAT)
   c) Rapid rabies enzyme immunodiagnosis (RREID)
   d) Rapid fluorescent focus inhibition test (RFFIT)

610. The sample preferred for diagnosis of clinical rabies is
   a) Saliva b) CSF
   c) Hair follicle d) Corneal tissue

611. Ante-mortem diagnosis of rabies can be made from the following sample
   a) Saliva b) Brain
   c) Urine d) Corneal tissue

612. Antigenic drift is common in the following disease
   a) Bovine leukemia
   b) Equine infectious anaemia
   c) Equine influenza
   d) All the above

613. The dose of equine rabies immunoglobulins for passive immunization is

a) 10 IU b) 20 IU
c) 30 IU d) 40 IU

614. The dose of human rabies immunoglobulins for passive immunization is

a) 10 IU b) 20 IU
c) 30 IU d) 40 IU

615. The number of subtypes of FMD virus prevalent worldwide are

a) 50 b) 60
c) 90 d) 80

616. Which one of the following host is a reservoir of rabies?

a) Monkey b) Jackel
c) Vampire bat d) All the above

617. Which one of the following has a long incubation period?

a) Johne's disease b) TSE
c) Bovine leukosis d) All the above

618. The dead end host for rabies is

a) Man b) Cattle
c) Horse d) All the above

619. Acute outbreaks of swine fever by virulent strains may cause

a) 100% mortality b) 50% mortality
c) 70% mortality d) None of the above

620. Subclinical rabies can occur in

a) Dog b) Cat
c) Both a and b d) Man

621. Hydrophobia is a sign in the following host

a) Horse b) Cattle
c) Man d) All the above

622. Photophobia is a sign in the following host

a) Man b) Cattle
c) Dog d) All the above

623. In FMD, the case- fatality in indigenous cattle is generally

a) 1 per cent
b) 40 per cent
c) 3-5 per cent
d) 20 per cent

624. Bellowing is a characteristic sign of rabies in

a) Dog
b) Sheep
c) Cattle
d) All the above

625. The primary vector involved in the transmission of African swine fever is

a) *Ornithodorus sp*
b) *Ixodes sp*
c) *Rhipicephalus sp*
d) All the above

626. In foot and mouth disease, the case- fatality in suckling calves may be

a) 10 per cent
b) 100 per cent
c) 50 per cent
d) 80 per cent

627. Colic is a characteristic sign of rabies in

a) Dog
b) Horse
c) Man
d) Pig

628. Which one of the following is resistant to rabies?

a) Lamb
b) Poultry
c) Calf
d) Skunk

629. African horse sickness virus is closely related to the virus of

a) Blue tongue
b) Hairy shaker disease
c) Both a and b
d) Bovine viral diarrhoea

630. The important source in the transmission of bovine leucosis is

a) Semen
b) Embryo
c) Blood
d) All the above

631. The reservoirs for African swine fever are

a) Feral pigs
b) Ticks
c) Both a and b
d) Earthworms

632. The number of serotypes of FMD virus prevalent worldwide are

a) 80
b) 3
c) 5
d) 7

633. Which one of the following clinical form is common in bovine leucosis?

a) Chronic b) Subacute
c) Virulent d) Peracute

634. In foot and mouth disease, the case- fatality in exotic cattle is

a) 20 per cent b) 80 per cent
c) 30 per cent d) 50 per cent

635. Which one of the following is true in immunity to natural infection by FMD?

a) Antibodies produced are serotype specific
b) Antibodies are cross protective to various serotypes and subtypes
c) Protective immunity is conferred for I year
d) All the above

636. Pig louse can mechanically transmit the following disease

a) Swine pox b) Hog cholera
b) Wart-hog disease d) Salmonellosis

637. The organ commonly affected in bovine leucosis is

a) Brain b) Liver
c) Spleen d) Lymph node

638. Biological transmission is not a feature in the following?

a) Equine encephalosis b) Louping-ill
c) Wart-hog disease d) Equine infectious anaemia

639. The reservoirs for swine fever are

a) Ticks b) Domestic pigs
c) Feral pigs d) Earthworms

640. African swine fever is transmitted by the method

a) Ingestion of meat scraps b) Ticks bite
c) Both a and b d) Inhalation

641. Digital hyperkeratosis is an important clinical feature of the following disease

a) Blue tongue b) Feline pan leukoaenia
c) Canine distemper d) Avian leukosis

642. Which one of the following is a list A disease classified by OIE?

a) Rinderpest b) CCPP
c) African horse sickness d) All the above

643. Purplish discolouration of the skin in swine fever is due to the following

a) Thrombocytopenia b) Vasculitis
c) Both a and b d) Leukopaenia

644. The pathogenic effect of bovine leucosis virus is

a) Leukopaenia b) Benign lymphocytosis
c) Malignant lymphocytosis d) Neutropaenia

645. Which one of the following is true for swine fever and African swine fever?

a) Both can be differentiated only by clinical signs.
b) Latent infection is the outcome of the both infections.
c) African swine fever is more severe than swine fever
d) All the above.

646. Malignant catarrhal fever is highly fatal in the following

a) Cattle b) Deer
c) Both a and b d) Sheep & goat

647. Trembling-ill in sheep may be predisposed by

a) Tick borne fever b) Tick pyaemia
c) Ehrlichiosis d) None of the above

648. African horse sickness is characterized by

a) Vascular leakage b) Thrombocytopaenia
c) Haemolysis d) None of the above

649. Bovine viral diaarhoea virus in cattle may potentiate pathogenicity of

a) PI-3 b) IBR virus
c) *Pasteurella* d) None of the above

650. Zebra markings in the large intestine are characteristic of the following

a) Rinderpest b) Foot and mouth disease
c) Johne's disease d) None of the above

651. The highly susceptible breed to canine distemper is
  a) Dolichocephalic breed b) German shepherd
  c) Labrador retriever d) Brachycephalic breed

652. In the diagnosis of *Microsporon* by woods lamp, yellowish green fluorescence emitted is due to the presence of the substance
  a) Tryphtophan b) Glycine
  c) Keratin d) None of the above

653. Difficulty in the control of equine infectious anaemia is due to
  a) Life-long viraemia in the affected animals
  b) Short period of immunity in vaccinated animals
  c) Multiple serotypes circulating in the field
  d) Hardy nature of the virus in the environment

654. Antigen -antibody complex in equine infectious anemia may lead to
  a) Glomerulitis b) Encephalitis
  c) Urticaria d) None of the above

655. Which one of the following features are noticed in equine infectious anemia?
  a) Vasculitis b) Oedema
  c) Haemolytic anaemia d) All the above

656. Canine parvovoiral infection causes immunodeficiency due to
  a) Destruction of neutrophils b) Destruction of CD4+ cells
  c) Protein deficiency d) Lymphoid cell depletion

657. Hair perforation test is employed in the diagnosis of
  a) Fungal infection b) Coccidioidomycosis
  c) Cryptococcosis d) Dermatophytosis

658. Pink colonies in Brilliant green agar are the characteristic diagnostic findings of
  a) Staphylococcosis b) Colibacillosis
  c) Streptococcosis d) Salmonellosis

659. Equine infectious anaemia is closely related to
  a) Feline infectious anaemia b) Bovine leukemia
  c) Chicken infectious anemia d) All the above

660. The disease caused by dermatophytes is called
    a) Ringworm
    b) Coccidioidomycosis
    c) Cryptococcosis
    d) Histoplasmosis

661. Canine distemper virus can effectively be disinfected in hospitals by
    a) 0.5 % Phenol
    b) Chloroform
    c) 5% Phenol
    d) 0.5% bleach

662. The primary method of transmission of the canine distemper virus in dogs is
    a) Cutaneous
    b) Ingestion
    c) Inhalation
    d) Congenital

663. In bovine leucosis, 90% of the cases are in
    a) Enzootic form
    b) Sporadic form
    c) Persistent form
    d) Epidemic form

664. 'Pink eye' refers to the following disease
    a) Marek's disease
    b) Infectious canine hepatitis
    c) Equine influenza
    d) None of the above

665. In FMD, foot lesions are generally severe in
    a) Cattle
    b) Goat
    c) Pig
    d) Sheep

666. Pseudoglanders refers to the disease
    a) Coccidiodomycosis
    b) Spororotrichosis
    c) Ulcerative lymphangitis
    d) Melioidosis

667. The breed which is at risk for the susceptibility to canine parvoviral enteritis is
    a) Rottweiler
    b) Dobermann pinscher
    c) Both a and b
    d) Cocker spaniel

668. Bovine papilloma virus-2 in cattle may cause
    a) Hepatitis
    b) Opthalmitis
    c) Haematuria
    d) All the above

669. Benign tuberculosis is common in

a) Cattle b) Man
c) Equines d) Pig

670. The signs of foot and mouth disease are generally mild in the following host

a) Buffaloe b) Pig
c) Sheep and goat d) Horse

671. In exotic cattle, rinderpest causes mortality up to

a) 90% b) 50 %
c) 10% d) 70%

672. Papillomatosis in horses result in the development of

a) Sarcoids b) Warts
c) Nodules d) Ulcers

673. 'Tinea' refers to the disease

a) Ringworm b) *Taenia solium* infection
c) Cestodiasis d) None of the above

674. In which one of the following disease, mortality is generally absent

a) Vesicular stomatitis b) FMD
c) Rinderpest d) MCF

675. In BVD, more than 90% of the cases are

a) Inapparent b) Clinical
c) Latent carriers d) Incubatory carriers

676. Bovine viral diarrhoea causes economic loss due to

a) Abortion b) Repeat breeding
c) Birth of weak calves d) All the above

677. Pseudo foot and mouth disease refers to the following disease

a) Vesicular exanthema b) Swine vesicular disease
c) Vesicular stomatitis d) None of the above

678. Ephemeral fever is transmitted by

a) *Culicoides sp* b) *Culex sp*
b) *Aedes sp.* d) All the above

679. The dermatophytes which is common in cattle is
   a) *T. verrucosum* b) T. mentagraphytes
   c) *M. gypseum* d) *M. nanum*

680. Enzootic bovine leucosis is common in the following age group of bovines
   a) Adults b) Less than 6 months old
   c) Above 6 months old d) None of the above

681. Oral form of canine papillomatosis is commonly seen in
   a) Young age b) Adults
   c) Females d) Males

682. Transovarian transmission is possible in
   a) Marek's disease b) IBD
   b) Fowl pox d) Infectious bronchitis

683. Blind layer is a feature in chickens infected with
   a) Avian encephalitis b) Egg drop syndrome-76
   c) Fowl pox d) Infectious bronchitis

684. Vaccination of cattle with modified live vaccines against IBR can result in
   a) Latent infection b) Abortion
   c) Transmission of the agent d) All the above

685. Vertical method of transmission in bovine leucosis is
   a) Congenital b) Transcolostral
   c) Transovarian d) All the above

686. Sporangia with endospores is a diagnostic stage in
   a) Tinea b) Coccidiodomycosis
   c) Spororotrichosis d) All the above

687. Prion infection in sheep results in
   a) Inflammation of neurons b) Degeneration of neurons
   c) Perivascular cuffing d) All the above

688. Ante-mortem diagnosis is difficult in the diagnosis of
   a) Rabies b) Scrapie
   c) Pseudorabies d) None of the above

689. Viral pneumonia is an infectious disease complex of calves managed under

a) Intensive system b) Extensive system
c) Semi-intensive system d) None of the above

690. Which one of the following form is common in bovine leucosis?

a) Classical enzootic form b) Sporadic form
c) Persistent form d) None of the above

691. The method of transmission in enzootic bovine leukosis is

a) Physical contact b) Ingestion
c) Vector bite d) All the above

692. Viral papillomatosis is common in the following host

a) Cattle b) Horse
c) Dog d) All the above

693. Vaccination against anaplasmosis is a risk factor in the transmission of

a) Tetanus b) Aspergillosis
c) Rinderpest d) Bovine leucosis

694. Favus cups are characteristic signs in the disease caused by *Trichophyton sp* in

a) Cattle b) Dog
c) Horse d) Bird

695. The diagnostic stage of fungus in ringworm is

a) Microconidia b) Arthrospores
c) Macroconidia d) Hyphae

696. Marbling of lymphnodes is characteristic of the following

a) Melioidosis b) Hog cholerea
c) Strangles d) Bovine leukosis

697. The media for identification of yeast form of the fungus is

a) Blood agar b) Sabaoraud's dextrose agar
c) Meat broth d) Nutrient agar

698. False strangles refers to the following disease
a) Ulcerative lymphangitis b) Histoplasmosis
c) Melioidosis d) None of the above

699. Sporotrichosis can be transmitted to horses by
a) Physical contact
b) Cat scratch
c) Contact with decayed plants
d) All the above

700. Oral form of papilloma are commonly seen in
a) Cattle b) Horse
c) Pig d) Dog

701. Intestinal spirochaetosis is caused by
a) *Leptospira* Pomona b) *L.* Tarassovi
c) *Borrelia theileri* d) *Brachyspira hyodysentriae*

702. The nerve involved in the paralysis due to Marek's disease is
a) Trigeminal nerve b) Optic nerve
c) Facial nerve d) Sciatic nerve

703. Which one of the following is a not a facultative intracellular agent?
a) *Listeria monocytogenes* b) *Brucella abortus*
c) *Salmonella* Typhimurium d) *M. bovis*

704. SMEDI is a syndrome in pigs caused by
a) *Brucella cholerae suis* b) Corona virus
c) *Listeria monocytogenes* d) Parvo virus

705. Which one of the following is not true to mycotoxicoses?
a) Non-antigenic b) Non-contagious
c) Non- immunogenic d) Infective

706. Feline distemper in cats is a synonym of
a) Cat pox b) Cat flu
c) Cat scratch fever d) Feline infectious peritonitis

707. The disease which can cause early abortion in cattle is
a) Brucellosis b) Campylobacteriosis
c) Q fever d) Listeriosis

708. Colibacillosis in calves commonly occurs in the age group of

a) > 1week
b) < 1 week
c) > 6months
d) > 1 month

709. The drug of choice for the treatment of Lyme disease is

a) Penicillin
b) Doxycycline
c) Ciprofloxacin
d) Erythromycin

710. Which one of the following fungal toxin is not hepatoxic?

a) Aflatoxin
b) Rubratoxin
c) Zearelenone
d) Sporidesmin

711. Quarantine refers to the physical separation of individuals which are

a) Diseased
b) Healthy
c) Recovered
d) Dead

712. Black quarters is caused by

a) *Clostridium chauvoi*
b) *Clostridium welchii*
c) Both a and b
d) *Clostridium septicum*

713. Erythema chronicum migrans (ECM) or Bull's eye is a sign of Lyme disease in

a) Dog
b) Cattle
c) Human
d) Poultry

714. Passive immunization with antitoxins against tetanus in sheep and horses can confer immunity for a period of

a) 7 day
b) 1 month
c) 14 days
d) 6 months

715. Transmissible gastroenteritis in pigs is caused by

a) *Brachyspira hyodysentriae*
b) Parvo virus
c) Corona virus
d) *S.* Cholerae suis

716. Which one of the following is a highly endemic in India?

a) Leptospirosis
b) Anthrax
c) Rabies
d) Brucellosis

717. Characteristic necropsy finding in sheep that died of enterotoxaemia due to *Clostridium perfringens* type D is

a) Hepatitis b) Lymph node enlargement
c) Pulpy kidney d) Myocarditis

718. Infectious bursal disease in chickens is caused by

a) Avibirna virus b) Avula virus
c) Paramyxo viridae d) Rubula virus

719. Coomb's test is generally employed in the diagnosis of

a) Leptospirosis b) Brucellosis
c) Anthrax d) Listeriosis

720. 'Sportsman posture' is a characteristic symptom observed in the following disease

a) Listeriosis b) Marek's disease
c) Pseudorabies d) Glassers disease

721. Which one of the following fungal toxin is not nephrotoxic?

a) Ochratoxin b) Oosporeine
c) Citrinin d) Ergotamine

722. Which one of the following is not a common agent in environmental mastitis?

a) *Streptococcus* dysagalactiae b) *Staphylococcus aureus*
c) *Streptococcus uberis* d) *E.coli*

723. The most common cause of food poisoning worldwide is

a) *E.coli* b) *S. Enteritidis*
c) *C. perfringens* type A d) *Y. enterocolitica*

724. The host in which the pathogen normally lives and multiplies is called

a) Latent carrier b) Reservoir
c) Persistent carrier d) Incubatory carrier

725. Aflatoxicosis in animals is caused by

a) *Aspergillus flavus* b) *A. parasiticus*
c) Both a and b d) *A. fumigatus*

726. Parvo virus in adult cattle causes

a) TGE
b) Abomasitis
c) Winter dysentry
d) Hepatitis

727. The route of transmission of *Brucella abortus* in animals and man is

a) Oral
b) Congenital
c) Mucosal
d) All the above

728. Winter dysentery in pigs is caused by

a) *Brachyspira hyodysentriae*
b) *Brachyspira pilosicoli*
c) Both a and b
d) Corona virus

729. The *Borrelia species* which affects livestock is

a) *B. theileri*
b) *B. coriaceae*
c) Both a and b
d) *B. burgdorferi*

730. In psittacosis, the elementary bodies of *Chlamydophila* can be identified by

a) Z-N technique
b) Gram's staining
c) Leishman staining
d) Modified Z-N test

731. Gas gangrene is caused by

a) *C. perfringens* type B
b) *Clostridium welchii*
c) *C. perfringens* type A
d) *Clostridium septicum*

732. The drug of choice in the treatment of leptospiraemia in the early stage is

a) Ciprofloxacin
b) Doxycycline
c) Dihydrostreptomycin
d) Amoxicillin

733. The methods used in the diagnosis of fowlpox is

a) Electron microscopy
b) Demonstration of intracytopathic inclusion bodies
c) Inoculation into CAM route of embryonated eggs
d) All the above

734. The most toxic and carcinogenic aflatoxin is

a) Aflatoxin G1
b) Aflatoxin B2
c) Aflatoxin M1
d) Aflatoxin B1

735. The common cause of death in patients affected with leptospirosis is
   a) Encephalitis b) Hepatic failure
   c) Haemolytic anaemia d) Renal failure

736. The following is a bacterium which does not possess cell wall
   a) *Mycoplasma bovis* b) *Streptococcus equi*
   c) *Actinomyces bovis* d) *E. coli*

737. Chondroid formation is a complication in horses of the disease
   a) Glanders b) Pseudostrangles
   c) Equine distemper d) Strangles

738. Gumboro disease causes high mortality in
   a) Pigeons b) Broilers
   c) Turkeys d) Layers

739. Carre's disease refers to
   a) Corona viral entertis b) Kennel cough
   c) Contagious canine hepatitis d) Canine distemper

740. BCG is a live attenuated vaccine consisting of
   a) *M. africanum* b) *M. tuberculosis*
   c) *M. microti* d) *M. bovis*

741. The disadvantage of rose Bengal plate agglutination test in the diagnosis of brucellosis is
   a) The test cannot detect only IgG antibodies.
   b) It cannot differentiate naturally infected and vaccinated animals.
   c) It shows cross reaction with *Salmonella* or *Yersinia* or *Escherchia.*
   d) All the above

742. Outbreak of encephalitis due to listeriosis commonly occurs after the feeding of
   a) Silage with pH>4.5 b) Silage with pH>3.0
   c) Silage with pH>2.5 d) Silage with pH>5.5

743. The species which is highly susceptible to aflatoxicosis is
   a) Ducklings b) Chicken
   c) Cattle d) Pig

744. 'False brush border' is a characteristic lesion in the large intestine of pigs infected by

a) *Brachyspira hyodysentriae* b) *Brachyspira pilosicoli*
c) Both a and b d) Corona virus

745. The Clostridial toxin employed in Nagler's reaction is

a) Alpha toxin b) Beta toxin
c) Gamma toxin d) Theta toxin

746. Which one of the following spirochaete is a facultative intracellular parasite?

a) *Borrelia burgdorferi* b) *Leptospira interrogans*
c) *Brachyspira hyodysentriae* d) All the above

747. Rubratoxin, a fungal toxin is produced by

a) *Penicillium rubram* b) *Penicillium purpurogenum*
c) Both a and b d) *Penicillium viridicatum*

748. Canine flu is caused by

a) Adeno virus b) Parvo virus
c) Morbilli virus d) Lyssa virus

749. Pox disease is mainly transmitted by arthropods in the following

a) Swinepox b) Horsepox
c) Horsepox d) Sheeppox

750. Swine erysipelas should be differentiated clinically from

a) Swinepox b) Swine fever
c) Salmonellosis d) All the above

751. Which one of the following is a category A bioterrorism agent?

a) *B. anthracis* b) *Francisella tularensis*
c) *Yersinia pestis* d) All the above

752. Tick borne fever in sheep has the following complication

a) Tick pyaemia b) Listeriosis
c) Joint-ill d) All the above

753. Which one of the following is an obligatory intracellular bacterium?

a) *Chlamydophila psittaci* b) *M. tuberculosis*
c) *Brucella suis* d) *Listeria* sp.

754. Ochratoxin and citrinin are the toxins produced by the fungi
    a) *Penicillium cyclopium*
    b) *Aspergillus ochraceus*
    c) *Penicillium viridicatum*
    d) All the above

755. Thrombocytopaenia is a feature of the following disease
    a) Plague
    b) Typhus fever
    c) Leptospirosis
    d) All the above

756. Very virulent IBD virus cause mortality in chickens which may be as high as
    a) 10-20 %
    b) 80-90 %
    c) 50-70 %
    d) 5-10 %

757. Which one of the following bacteria is excreted through milk?
    a) *Brucella melitensis*
    b) *Listeria monocytogenes*
    c) *Mycobacterium bovis*
    d) All the above

758. The common clinical sign of borreliosis in poultry is
    a) Fever
    b) Arthritis
    c) Anaemia
    d) None of the above

759. Septic abortion in sheep and goats is caused by
    a) *Chlamydophila abortus*
    b) *Chlamydophila caviae*
    c) *Chlamydophila psittaci*
    d) *Chlamydophila pneumonia*

760. The reservoir for *Leptospira* Hardjo is
    a) Pig
    b) Dog
    c) Cattle
    d) Horse

761. Which one of the following does not produce the mycotoxin zearelenone?
    a) *Fusarium graminearum*
    b) *Fusarium roseum*
    c) *Fusarium tricinctum*
    d) All the above

762. Hard pad disease in dogs is caused by
    a) Adeno virus
    b) Parvo virus
    c) Morbilli virus
    d) Lyssa virus

763. Yellow lamb disease is caused by
    a) *Clostridium septicum*
    b) *Clostridium welchii*
    c) *C. perfringens* type A
    d) *C. perfringens* type C

764. Avian diphtheria is caused by

a) *Trichomonas gallinae* b) *Candida albicans*
c) Avipox virus d) Corona virus

765. *Chalmydophila psiattaci* genotype A affects specifically

a) Parrots b) Pigeons
c) Turkeys d) Ducks

766. Typhus fever is caused by

a) *Rickettsia prowasekii* b) *Rickettsia typhi*
c) Both a and b d) *R. conori*

767. Weil-Felix test is employed in the diagnosis of

a) *Ehrlichia sp* b) *Rickettsia sp*
c) *Chlamydophila sp* d) *Anaplasma sp*

768. In avian flu, birds act as mixing vessels for reassortment of

a) H2N2 b) H5N1
c) H1N1 d) H3N8

769. Kyasanur forest disease is a mosquito borne flavi viral disease of man transmitted from

a) Birds b) Monkeys
c) Pigs d) Bats

770. Which one of the following is not a lesion of IBD?

a) Haemorrhage at the junction of proventriculus and gizzard
b) Enlarged and oedematous bursa in acute stage of disease
c) Atropy of bursa in chronic stage of disease
d) Haemorrhage in the villi of proventriculus

771. Jenner's pox is noticed in

a) Pigs b) Horse
c) Cow d) Chicken

772. Old dog encephalitis occurs due to the persistence of the virus in the following disease

a) Rubarth's disease b) Rabies
c) Canine distemper d) Leptospirosis

773. The reservoir for infectious canine hepatitis is

a) Bats b) Rodents
c) Fox d) Rabbits

774. Gray eye or fish eye is a characteristic lesion in the following disease

a) Marek's disease b) Equine influenza
c) Morexellosis d) ICH

775. Swine erysipelas results in high mortality in the following

a) Asiatic pigs b) Wild pigs
c) Turkey d) African pigs

776. Which one of the following is not a strain of IBD virus?

a) Mild strain b) Intermediate strain
c) Mass d) Intermediate and hot strain

777. The reservoir for Lyme disease is

a) White tailed deer b) White footed mouse
c) Both a and b d) Bats

778. 'Gold medallion' lesion is a hyper reflective area in the eye which is characteristic of

a) Parvo viral enteritis b) Rota viral infection
c) Canine distemper d) Kennel cough

779. 'Figure of eight knot' is the microscopic appearance of

a) *P. multocida* b) *Bordetella bronchiseptica*
c) *Yersinia enterocolitica* d) *Clostridium septicum*

780. Wooden cattle is caused by

a) *Actinomyces bovis* b) *Bacillus anthracis*
c) *Clostridium tetani* d) *Actinobcaillus lignieresi*

781. 'Saw horse' appearance is a characteristic sign of the disease

a) Anthrax b) Rabies
c) Tetanus d) Actinomycosis

782. 'Medusa head' or 'ground glass' appearance in blood agar is characteristic of the bacterial agent

a) *Bacillus anthracis* b) *L. interrogans*
c) *Listeria monocytogenes* d) *Chlamydophila psittaci*

783. The virus of infectious canine hepatitis is antigenically related to the canine virus of

a) Infectious laryngotracheitis b) Leptospirosis
c) Canine influenza d) Fox encephalitis

784. Which one of the following is called as Kirkuth's disease?

a) Fowlpox b) Horsepox
c) Swinepox d) Sheeppox

785. Polioencephalomalacia of temporal lobes in canine distemper results in

a) Chewing gum seizures b) Chorea
c) Myoclonus d) Encephalitis

786. Which one of the following produces the mycotoxin, tricothecenes?

a) *Fusarium graminearum* b) *Fusarium roseum*
c) *Fusarium tricinctum* d) *F. moniliformae*

787. The OIE recommended serological test in the diagnosis of IBD in chickens is

a) HI b) AGID
c) IFA d) All the above

788. The method of transmission of black quarters may be

a) Endogenous b) Exogenous
c) Both a and b d) Physical injury

789. 'Red water' is a disease caused by

a) *Leptospira* Hardjo b) L. Icterohaemorrhagiae
c) *Clostridium haemolyticum* d) *Clostridium tetani*

790. Which one of the following is called as catpox?

a) Monkeypox b) Vaccinia
c) Cowpox d) Camelpox

791. Dogs act as reservoirs for the following serovar of *Leptospira*

a) L. Canicola b) L. Bataviae
c) Both a and b d) L. Pomona

792. Lemon shaped spores are characteristic of the following bacteria

a) *C. tetani* b) *C. perfringens*
c) *C. chauvoi* d) *Clostridium septicum*

793. Pasture fever in cattle is caused by

a) *Anapalsma marginale* b) *Anapalsma centrale*
c) *Anapalsma phagocytophilum* d) *Coxiella burnetti*

794. The disadvantage of vaccination with RB 51 strain against brucellosis is

a) It may still cause disease in human
b) The strain is rifampin resistant
c) It results in low protective titre
d) All the above

795. Ergot toxins are produced by

a) *Pithomyces chartarum* b) *Penicillium viridicatum*
c) *Fusarium tricinctum* d) *Claviceps pupuria*

796. Marek's disease in poultry causes

a) Fowl paralysis b) Neural lymphoma
c) Skin leukosis d) All the above

797. The potential reservoir for *Leptospira* Icterohaemorrhagiae is

a) Bats b) Birds
c) Rodents d) Pigs

798. The characteristic sign of typhus fever is

a) Epistaxis b) Melena
c) Centripetal rash d) Fever

799. The age at which vaccination against brucellosis in cattle is recommended is

a) 1-2 month b) 3-4 months
c) 5-8 months d) 2-3 months

800. Which one of the following does not favour mycotoxin production?

a) Increased O_2 b) 70% Rh
c) 52-55 % moisture d) 20-25°C temperature

801. Disseminated intravascular coagulation (DIC) is a feature of the disease

a) Plague b) Salmonellosis
c) Chlamydophilosis d) All the above

802. The OIE recommended serological test in the diagnosis of Newcastle disease in chickens is

a) HI b) AGID
c) VNT d) Immunoflourescence

803. Which one of the following pox disease is not zoonotic?

a) Contagious ecthyma b) Pseudocow pox
c) Buffalopox d) Sheeppox

804. Floppy broiler syndrome is caused by

a) Alpha herpes virus b) Type C retro virus
c) Onco virus d) Gallid herpes virus

805. Lyme disease in dogs is characterized by

a) Arthritis b) Edema
c) Fever d) All the above

806. Rodents act as reservoirs for the following serovar of *Leptospira*

a) *L.* Icterhaemorrhagiae b) *L.* Ballum
c) Both a and b d) *L.* Pomona

807. In epidemic typhus, development of centripetal rashes on the body is due to

a) Delayed hypersensitivity b) Vasculitis
c) Allergic reaction d) All the above

808. The highly susceptible host for avian mycoplasmosis is

a) Turkey b) Pheasants
c) Game birds d) Chicken

809. The reservoir for cowpox is

a) Birds b) Rodents
c) Pigs d) Bats

810. Flabby udder mastitis in cattle is caused by

a) *S. aureus* b) *L.* Hardjo
c) *Listeria monocytogenes* d) *E.coli*

811. Canine Lyme disease is caused by

a) *B. anserina* b) *Borrelia burgdorferi*
c) *Borrelia sp.* d) *Borrelia recurrentis*

812. Beta haemolysis is characteristic of the following agent

a) *Sreptococcus pneumoniae* b) *Staphylococcus aureus*
c) Both a and b d) *C. pseudotuberculosis*

813. The chronic infectious fatal gastrointestinal disease in ruminants characterized by progressive emaciation and diarrhea is

a) Johne's disease b) Tuberculosis
c) Bovine viral diarrhoea d) Rota viral enteritis

814. The highly infective and insidious disease in ruminants characterized by granular enteritis is

a) Parauberculosis b) Tuberculosis
c) Salmonellosis d) Rota viral enteritis

815. Latent infection is the outcome of infection in the following disease

a) Marek's disease b) ILT
c) Both a and b d) IBD

816. Sheep and goat pox in systemic form commonly result in

a) Bronchopneumonia b) Enteritis
c) Hepatitis d) Lameness

817. Catarrhal fever of sheep is caused by

a) Orbi virus b) Morbilli virus
c) Parapox virus d) Aptha virus

818. Ascoli's test is the serological test used in the diagnosis of

a) Anthrax b) Tuberculosis
c) IBD d) Quarter-ill

819. Necrotic enteritis in chickens is caused by

a) *Clostridium novy* b) *C. perfringens* type A
c) *Clostridium haemolyticum* d) *Clostridium septicum*

820. Colourless non-hamolytic and dew drop like colonies are characteristic of the following bacteria

a) *S. aureus* b) *Brucella abortus*
c) *Salmonella* Dublin d) *E.coli*

821. RB51 strain is preferred for vaccination against brucellosis for the following reason

a) It can be used in pregnant cows
b) Male calves can be vaccinated using this strain
c) Differentiation of naturally infected and vaccinated cows is possible.
d) All the above

822. Etiology of bacillary haemoglobinuria in cattle is

a) *Leptospira* Hardjo
b) *C. perfringens* type A
c) *Clostridium haemolyticum*
d) *Clostridium septicum*

823. Orf is also referred to as

a) Scabby mouth b) Sore mouth
c) Both a and b d) Spurious pox

824. Emetic syndrome in pigs is caused by the fungal toxin

a) Zeareleneone b) Ochratoxin
c) Tricothecenes d) Citrinin

825. Bipolar rods are characteristic of the following bacteria

a) *P. multocida* b) *Yersinia pestis*
c) Both a and b d) *Clostridium septicum*

826. Chronic respiratory disease in chickens is caused by

a) *M. gallisepticum* b) *M. synoviae*
c) *M. meleagridis* d) *M. iowae*

827. Pig act as reservoirs for the following serovar of *Leptospira*

a) L. Icterhaemorrhagiae b) L. Australis
c) L. Gripphotyphosa d) L. Pomona

828. Which one of the following is a mechanism in the pathogenesis of mycotoxicosis?
   a) Reduced nutrient absorption and impaired metabolism
   b) Alterations in the endocrine and exocrine systems
   c) Suppression of the immune system
   d) All the above

829. Terminal dry gangrene in cattle is caused by the fungal toxin
   a) Ergotamine   b) Ergometrine
   c) Both a and b   d) Sporidesmin

830. 'Wooden horse posture' is a complication due to bloat of the disease
   a) Actinomycosis   b) Tetanus
   c) Black quarters   d) Anthrax

831. 'Ring sore' in cow is caused by
   a) FMD   b) Buffalopox
   c) Dermatophytosis   d) Pseudocowpox

832. Which one of the following is not associated with severity of the chronic respiratory disease in chickens?
   a) Newcastle disease   b) Colibacillosis
   c) Infectious bronchitis   d) Salmonellosis

833. CAMP test is used in the diagnosis of
   a) *C. tetani*   b) *Clostridium welchii*
   c) *C. perfringens*   d) *Clostridium botulinum*

834. 'Box car appearance' in Gram's staining is characteristic of the following bacteria
   a) *Actinomyces bovis*   b) *Dermatophilus congolensis*
   c) *B. anthracis*   d) *Streptococcus equi*

835. The nerve involved in the transmission of nervous form of listeriosis is
   a) Vestibular nerve   b) Olfactory nerve
   c) Trigeminal nerve   d) Sciatic nerve

836. 'Pump handle breathing' is characteristic of the following disease
   a) Infectious laryngotracheitis   b) Chronic respiratory disease
   c) Pneumonic pasteurellosis   d) Tetanus

837. The positive titre for bovine brucellosis in endemic area is
 a) 1:10 b) 1:20
 c) 1:40 d) 1:80

838. Sore muzzle of sheep is a synonym of
 a) Peste des petits ruminants b) Sheep pox
 c) Orf d) Bluetongue

839. Breast bone fever or pigeon fever is a disease of horse caused by
 a) *S. aureus* b) *Actinobacillus equilii*
 c) *S. equi* d) *C. peudotuberculosis*

840. Which one of the following is the clinical sign of mycoplasmosis in turkeys?
 a) Conjunctivitis b) Closed eyelids
 c) Infraorbital sinus swelling d) All the above

841. Which one of the following fungus causes photosensitization in sheep?
 a) *Pithomyces chartarum* b) *Penicillium rubrum*
 c) *Claviceps pupurea* d) None of the above

842. Systemic form of pox is more common in the following disease
 a) Sheeppox b) Goatpox
 c) Contagious ecthyma d) All the above

843. Which one of the following is an oestrogenic mycotoxin affecting pigs?
 a) Zearelenone b) Ochratoxin
 c) Aflatoxin d) T-2 toxin

844. Natural service is an important method in the transmission of brucellosis in
 a) Pigs b) Cattle
 c) Bufffaloe d) All the above

845. Haemorrhagic necrocolitis in calves, lambs and foals is caused by
 a) *Clostridium perfringens* type B
 b) *C. perfringens* type D
 c) *Clostridium haemolyticum*
 d) *Clostridium septicum*

846. The group which is at risk of contracting brucellosis is
   a) Breeding animals b) Young calves
   c) 6 month old calves d) All the above

847. Zearelenone, a mycotoxin in pigs causes
   a) Vulval oedema b) Hepatitis
   c) Nephritis d) Endometritis

848. The selective medium used for the diagnosis of *Bacillus anthracis* is
   a) PLET b) Nutrient agar
   c) Robertson cooked medium d) Egg yolk agar

849. Avian distemper in chickens is caused by
   a) Avula virus b) Rubula virus
   c) Paramyxo virus d) Orthomyxo virus

850. Which one of the following is not a clinical sign of tetanus?
   a) Prolapse of nictitating membrane
   b) Pump handle tail
   c) Trismus
   d) Flaccid paralysis

851. All pathogenic *Leptospira* are classified into the following biospecies
   a) *L. interrogans* b) *L. biflexa*
   c) *L. Pomona* d) None of the above

852. The type of vaccine used in the control of sheeppox and goatpox is
   a) Live attenuated b) Killed
   c) Toxoid d) Genetic

853. The following is the reservoir for *C. chauvoi* spores
   a) Liver b) GI tract
   c) Both a and b d) Kidney

854. *Brucella* causes abortion in pregnant cows due to the presence of the following substance in placenta
   a) Polyhydric alcohol b) Enzymes
   c) Erythritol d) Amniotic protein

855. The sign of *M. synoviae* in chickens is
   a) Joint swelling b) Pale comb
   c) Urate droppings d) All the above

856. In botulism death occurs due to
   a) Respiratory paralysis b) Asphyxiation
   c) Both a and b d) Spastic paralysis

857. Air sacculitis is characteristic of the following disease
   a) *M. gallisepticum* b) *M. synoviae*
   c) S. Pullorum d) *P. multocida*

858. Development of oedema in anthrax is due to the release of following toxic factor
   a) Adenylate cyclase b) Aggressine
   c) Lethal factor d) Zinc metallo protein

859. Which one of the following is a contagious disease?
   a) Candidiasis b) Aspergillosis
   c) Histoplasmosis d) Dermatophilosis

860. Which one of the following is not a synonym of Newcastle disease?
   a) Avian pneumoencephalitis b) Avian distemper
   c) Fowl paralysis d) Pseudo-fowl plague

861. Case-fatality may reach higher in the following pox disease
   a) Cowpox b) Pseudocowpox
   c) Sheep pox d) All the above

862. Which one of the following is not a clinical feature of bluetongue in sheep?
   a) Abortion b) Bronchopneumonia
   c) Dummy lambs d) Vesicles on lips

863. One of the most common causative agents of joint-ill in foals is
   a) *Actinobacillus equuli* b) *S. aureus*
   c) *Fusobacterium necrophorum* d) *Mycoplasma*

864. Acute and fatal anaplasmosis can occur in the following
   a) Calves b) Suckling calves
   c) Lambs d) Adult Cattle

865. Which one of the following mycotoxin causes facial eczema in sheep?

a) Zearelenone b) Ochratoxin
c) Aflatoxin d) Sporidesmin

866. The sign of *M. synoviae* in chickens is

a) Sinusitis b) Tracheitis
c) Air sacculitis d) All the above

867. Complication in tick borne fever is commonly due to

a) Staphylococcal pyaemia b) Brucellosis
c) Listeriosis d) Pasteurellosis

868. The number of pathotypes of IBD virus is

a) One b) Two
c) Three d) Four

869. Which one of the following is not a common feature of aspergillosis in cattle?

a) Abortion
b) Mastitis
c) Granulomatous pneumonia
d) Enteritis

870. The disease which is transmitted by cat scratch is

a) *Sporotrichus schenkii* b) *Bartonella henslae*
c) *P. multocida* type A & C d) All the above

871. Eschar-like lesion is characteristic of the disease

a) Anthrax b) Plaque
c) Epidemic typhus d) Rickettsial pox

872. The reservoir of *Coccidioides immitis* is

a) Pigeons b) Rabbits
c) Rodents d) Water birds

873. The method not useful in the diagnosis of mycotoxicosis is

a) HPLC b) TLC
c) ELISA d) PCR

874. The drug of choice for avian mycoplasmosis is

a) Tylosin b) Tetracyclins
c) Amoxicillin d) Enrofloxacins

875. Flaccid paralysis which occurs in botulism is due to

a) Inhibition of Ach b) Inhibition of GABA
c) Inhibition of glycine d) None of the above

876. The vector most commonly involved in the transmission of bluetongue in sheep is

a) *Culicoides variipennis* b) *Melophagus ovinus*
c) Tabanus d) *Aedes sp*

877. Miliary brucellosis is common in the host

a) Pigs b) Mares
c) Sheep d) Dogs

878. Both papular and nodular forms are seen in the following pox disease

a) Sheeppox b) Cowpox
c) Goatpox d) Swinepox

879. Tetanus which occurs by transmission of spores via umbilicus of calves is

a) Idiopathic tetanus b) Puerperal tetanus
c) Tetanus neonatorum d) None of the above

880. Latency is the outcome of the following disease

a) Salmonellosis b) Brucellosis
c) Both a and b d) None of the above

881. 'Horse shoe' like spores are characteristic in the diagnosis of

a) Big head b) Tetanus
c) Braxy d) Bacillary haemoglobinuria

882. Absence of rigor mortis in anthrax is due to the release of following factor

a) Oedema factor b) Protective factor
c) Lethal factor d) All the above

883. The causative agent of joint-ill in calves is

a) *C. pyogenes* b) *Staphylococcus aureus*
c) *Fusobacterium necrophorum* d) All the above

884. The positive titre for bovine brucellosis in non-endemic area is

a) 1:40 b) 1:20
c) 1:10 d) 1:80

885. Which one of the following pathotype of IBD virus is velogenic viscerotropic?

a) Doyle's form b) Beaudette's form
c) Hitchner's form d) Komarov's form

886. Which one of the following is not a clinical sign of botulism?

a) Prolapse of third eyelid b) Ptosis
c) Dropping of jaw d) Flaccid paralysis

887. The selective medium used for the diagnosis of *M. bovis* is

a) Lowenstein Jensen Medium
b) Robertson meat broth
c) Nutrient agar
d) Blood agar

888. Caseous lymphadenitis is a bacterial disease of

a) Sheep b) Cattle
c) Pig d) All the above

889. Ulcerative lymphangitis in horses is characterized by the inflammation of lymph nodes most commonly on

a) Head b) Upper limb
c) Inguinal area d) Lower limb

890. 'Wasp-waist' appearance is characteristic in the diagnosis of

a) *C. tetani* b) *Clostridium welchii*
c) *C. oedematiens* d) *Clostridium botulinum*

891. Which one of the following is a method in the control of mycotoxicosis ?

a) Addition of additives like propionic acid

b) Addition of absorbents like bentonites in the feed
c) Increasing dietry levels of protein, energy and antioxidants
d) All the above

892. 'Stone pox' is generally referred to as
a) Sheep b) Cattle
c) Buffalo d) Goat

893. In tetanus death occurs due to
a) Renal failure b) Respiratory failure
c) Cardiac myositis d) Oedema

894. The sample commonly used for the isolation of NDV is
a) Faeces b) Allantoic fluid
c) Ocular discharge d) Amniotic fluid

895. Abortion is not a common feature of brucellosis in the following species
a) Equine b) Sheep
c) Pigs d) Human

896. In sheep and goats, *Corynebacterium pseudotuberculosis* causes the disease called
a) Ulcerative lymphangitis b) Breast bone fever
c) Ulcerative cellulitis d) Caseous lymphadenitis

897. Seven day fever is a synonym of the disease
a) Brucellosis b) Leptospirosis
c) Ephemeral fever d) Anthrax

898. Lamb dysentery is caused by
a) *Clostridium perfringens* type D b) *C. perfringens* type B
c) *Clostridium perfringens* type C d) *Clostridium novy*

899. Preiz-Nocard bacillus is commonly known as
a) *Malleomyces mallei* b) *Burkholderia pseudomallei*
c) *Dichelobacter nodosus* d) *C. pseudotuberculosis*

900. The complications of orf in sheep is
a) Cutaneous myiasis b) Dermatophilosis
c) Staphylococcosis d) All the above

901. Raspberry spleen is characteristic of the following disease

a) Swine fever
b) Leptospirosis
c) Bovine leukosis
d) Anthrax

902. 'Big head' is a disease in livestock caused by

a) *Clostridium perfringens* type B
b) *Clostridium novy A*
c) *C. septicum*
d) *Clostridium novy B*

903. Paratuberculosis infects cattle and buffalo at the age of

a) 3 months
b) 1 month
c) 6 months
d) Above 2 years

904. Tetanus which occurs by transmission of spores via birth canal in cows is called

a) Idiopathic tetanus
b) Puerperal tetanus
c) Tetanus neonatorum
d) None of the above

905. Which one of the following is called fowl plague?

a) ILT
b) Avian flu
c) IBD
d) Newcastle disease

906. The virulent factors of *M. tuberculosis* is

a) Cord factor
b) Sulfolipds
c) Glycolipds
d) All the above

907. The selective medium used for the diagnosis of *Clostridium tetani* is

a) Blood agar
b) Robertson meat broth
c) Nutrient agar
d) Egg yolk agar

908. Tennis racket or drumstick appearance is characteristic of the following bacteria

a) *C. tetani*
b) *Clostridium welchii*
c) *C. oedematiens*
d) *Clostridium septicum*

909. Which one of the following type of avian influenza virus affects all species?

a) Type A
b) Type B
c) Type C
d) All the above

910. The first bacterium to be observed under microscope is

a) *B. anthracis* b) *C. tetani*
c) *Salmonella* d) *Streptococcus*

911. The number of 'H' subtypes of highly pathogenic avian influenza virus is

a) 2 or 3 b) 5 or 7
c) 7 or 9 d) All the above

912. Three day fever in cattle is caused by

a) *B. abortus* b) *L. Hardjo*
c) *Ephemero virus* d) *Aptha virus*

913. Calf-hood vaccination is carried out for the following disease

a) FMD b) Haemorrhagic septicaemia
c) Brucellosis d) Johne's disease

914. Sour crop in chickens is caused by

a) *Trichophyton gallinae* b) *Trichomonas.gallinae*
c) *Candida albicans* d) *Cryptococcus neoformans*

915. Enterotoxaemia in lambs is predisposed by

a) Strongyloidosis b) Cysticercosis
c) Moneziasis d) Haemonchosis

916. Histoplasmosis is a contagious disease in the following species

a) Cattle b) Dog
c) Both a and b d) Horse

917. Hjarre's disease or coligranuloma in poultry is caused by

a) Verotoxic *E. coli* b) Cytonecrotoxic *E. coli*
c) Enterotxic *E. coli* d) Septicaemic *E. coli*

918. The selective medium used in the culture of *Leptospira* is

a) Lowenstein Jensen Medium
b) Robertson meat broth
c) EMJH medium
d) Egg yolk agar

919. Currently circulating subtypes of influenza virus of animals in human are

a) H1N1 b) H5N1
c) H3N2 d) All the above

920. Chronic form of overeating disease is common in

a) Sheep b) Lambs
c) Goats d) Kids

921. The following are the synonyms of candidiasis

a) Moniliasis b) Thrush
c) Crop mycosis d) All the above

922. Septicaemic *E.coli* in livestock causes the following disease

a) Pneumonia b) Meningitis
c) Navel-ill d) All the above

923. Ephemeral fever is also referred to as

a) Lazyman disease b) Dragon boat disease
c) Tongue fever d) All the above

924. Which one of the following toxins is involved in the pathogenesis of black quarters?

a) Necrotoxin b) Haemolysin
c) Both a and b d) Epsilon

925. 'Pink eye' in horses is caused by

a) *Morexella sp.* b) EHV-1
c) Orthomyxo virus d) *Leptospira*

926. In black quarters, death occurs due to

a) Renal failure b) Respiratory arrest
c) Cardiac myositis d) Gas formation

927. Terminal dry gangrene is a clinical feature in the following disease

a) Colibacillosis b) Acute salmonellosis
c) Chronic salmonellosis d) Septicaemic colibcaillosis

928. Bluetongue in sheep is most commonly transmitted by

a) *Culex* sp b) *Aedes* sp
c) Biting midges d) *Anapheles* sp

929. Thin ewe syndrome is caused by
   a) *M. paratuberculosis*
   b) *B. ovis*
   c) *C. pseudotuberculosis*
   d) *M. tuberculosis*

930. Enterotoxigenic *E.coli* in livestock causes the following disease
   a) Pneumonia
   b) Diarrhoea
   c) Haemorrhagic colitis
   d) All the above

931. 'Antigenic drift' and 'shift' are common in the following virus
   a) HPAI
   b) Type B influenza
   c) Type C influenza
   d) None of the above

932. Tuberculosis is characterized by the development of
   a) Oedema
   b) Gangrene
   c) Caseous necrosis
   d) Emphysema

933. The factors of the anthrax bacilli which produce toxic effects in the host are
   a) Oedema factor
   b) Protective factor
   c) Lethal factor
   d) All the above

934. MTBC is a complex that includes the following bacteria
   a) *M. bovis*
   b) *M. tuberculosis*
   c) *M. microti*
   d) All the above

935. Enterotoxaemia in adult goats is predominantly characterized by
   a) Diarrhoea
   b) Nervous signs
   c) Both a and b
   d) Renal failure

936. Watery mouth disease in pigs is caused by the following strain of *E.coli*
   a) Cytonecrotoxin
   b) Septicaemic
   c) Verotoxin
   d) Enterotoxin

937. Oedema of lips, gums and tongue of sheep is characteristic of the disease
   a) Bluetongue
   b) Lumpy skin disease
   c) Scabby mouth
   d) Sheep pox

938. Tubercle bacilli in milk can be destroyed by the following method
   a) Pasteurization b) Boiling for 30 min
   c) Both a and b d) Heating for 30 min

939. 'Black disease' in livestock is caused by
   a) *Clostridium welchii* b) *Clostridium novy A*
   c) *C. perfringens* type A d) *Clostridium novy B*

940. The routes of infection by *M. bovis* are
   a) Respiratory b) Oral
   c) Congenital d) All the above

941. Lamb-hood vaccination is carried out for the following disease
   a) Tuberculosis b) Haemorrhagic septicaemia
   c) Brucellosis d) Johne's disease

942. The reservoirs of avian flu are
   a) Wild water fowls b) Turkeys
   c) Pond herons d) Pigs

943. The organs affected in miliary tuberculosis is
   a) Lungs b) Bones
   c) Kidney d) All the above

944. Toxoids vaccines are employed in the control of
   a) *Clostridium perfringens* type B
   b) *Clostridium botulinum*
   c) *C. perfringens* type D
   d) All the above

945. The protein derivative derived from extracts of broth cultures of *M. tuberculosis* which elicits delayed typed hypersensitivity is
   a) Tuberculin b) Sulfolipds
   c) Glycoside d) Mycolic acid

946. Paired sera samples are collected in the disease diagnosis at the interval of
   a) 2-3 weeks b) 1-2 weeks
   c) 3 months d) 6 months

947. The most susceptible host of Johne's disease is

a) Cattle
b) Sheep
c) Pig
d) Goat

948. 'Pink eye' in cattle is caused by

a) *Morexella bovis*
b) BHV-1
c) OHV-2
d) Leptospirosis

949. Which one of the following breed is less susceptible to the disease bluetongue?

a) Merino
b) Asiatic breed
c) European breed
d) Dorset

950. Tetanus which occurs by ingestion of spores in the feed is called

a) Idiopathic tetanus
b) Puerperal tetanus
c) Tetanus neonatorum
d) None of the above

951. Avian flu is most commonly transmitted by the following route?

a) Faeco-oral
b) Respiratory
c) Vertical
d) All the above

952. Stress proteins are the virulent factors produced by

a) *Brucella sp.*
b) *Mycobacterium sp.*
c) Both a and b
d) *Bacillus sp.*

953. Enterotoxaemia in ruminants is clinically characterized by

a) Enteritis
b) Encephalitis
c) Both a and b
d) Nervous signs

954. The *Clostridium* species causing inflammation of the abomasal wall in sheep is

a) *Clostridium welchii*
b) *Clostridium novy A*
c) *Clostridium septicum*
d) *Clostridium novy B*

955. The terminal spores of *C. tetani* give the characteristic appearance of

a) Dumb bell appearance
b) Box car appearance
c) Drumstick appearance
d) Pallisade appearance

956. Heat shock protein (HSP) is a virulent factor which helps in the survival of

a) *Brucella* b) *Leptospira*
c) *Salmonella* d) All the above

957. Avian encephalitis generally occurs at the age of

a) 1-3 weeks b) < 20 weeks
c) >20 weeks d) 52 weeks

958. Paired sera samples are collected in the disease diagnosis to identify

a) Per acute infection b) Acute infection
c) Current infection d) Chronic infection

959. The most common manifestation of bovine actinomycosis seen in the bones of the head is

a) Non- suppurative osteomyelitis
b) Suppurative osteomyelitis
c) Osteoblastosis
d) Discospondylitis

960. In Pulpy kidney disease, the potency of epsilon toxin is increased by

a) Kappa toxin b) Lambda toxin
c) Pepsin d) All the above

961. The breed which is highly susceptible for coccidiodomycosis in dog is

a) Pointer b) Boxer
c) Non-decriptive d) Bull

962. The site of carrying out tuberculin test in poultry is

a) Comb b) Wattle
c) Wing web d) Thigh region

963. Vaccines against anthrax usually contain non-encapsulated

a) Ames strain b) Sterne strain
c) Vollum strain d) Cotton strain

964. "Tetaniferic regions" have the following type of soil favouring anaerobes

a) Sandy b) Alkaline
c) Clay d) Acidic

965. Guttural mycosis in horses is caused by

a) *Penicillium rubrum* b) *Pithomyces chartarum*
c) *A. fumigatus* d) *Fusarium roseum*

966. The origin of tumor cells in chickens affected with Marek's disease is

a) Myeloid cells b) Macrophages
c) B -cells d) T-cells

967. The first bacterium used in the preparation of attenuated strain is

a) *B. anthracis* b) *P. multocida*
c) *Salmonella* d) *E.coli*

968. Which one of the following *Salmonella* is transmitted by consumption by meat?

a) *Salmomella* Typhimurium b) *Salmonella* Dublin
c) *Salmonella* Pullorum d) *S.* Enteritidis

969. 'Bicycle leg movements' are characteristic of the following disease

a) Avian leukosis b) Marek's disease
c) Hypovitaminosis d) Avian encephalitis

970. The principle of intradermal test in the diagnosis of paratuberculosis is

a) Delayed hypersensitivity b) Immediate hypersensitivity
c) Anphylaxis d) Cellular infiltration

971. The virulence factor of *P.multocida* which is toxic to respiratory tract epithelial cells of cattle is

a) Lipopolysaccharide b) Leukotoxin
c) OMP d) Capsular antigen

972. Oedema disease in pigs is caused by the following strain of *E.coli*

a) Cytonecrotoxin b) Leukotoxin
c) Verotoxin d) Enterotoxin

973. Bacillary white diarrhoea in chicks is caused by

a) *Salmomella* Gallinarum b) *Salmonella* Arizonae
c) *Salmonella* Pullorum d) *S.* Enteritidis

974. Which one of the following is not a syndrome or sign of leptospirosis in livestock?

a) Milk drop syndrome b) Moon blindness
c) Weak calf syndrome d) Summer mastitis

975. The OIE recommended confirmatory serological test in the diagnosis of brucellosis is

a) CFT b) AGID
c) RBPT d) PCR

976. The positive titre for leptospirosis in animals is generally

a) 1:100 b) 1:50
c) 1:200 d) 1:400

977. The disease or sign caused by *P. multocida* in rabbits is

a) Pneumonia b) Atropic rhinitis
c) Arthritis d) Snuffles

978. Which one of the following is a not a potent immunosuppressive agent?

a) Aflatoxin b) Ochratoxin
c) T-2 toxin d) Citrinin

979. 'Wattle cholera' in chicken refers to pasteurellosis in

a) Acute stage b) Chronic stage
c) Per acute stage d) Septicaemic stage

980. '2 Mercapto -ethanol' test used in brucellosis differentiates

a) Acute and chronic infections
b) Per acute and acute forms
c) Clinical and subclinical forms
d) None of the above

981. Fistulous withers in horses is caused by the associated effect of

a) *Brucella abortus* b) *Actinomyces bovis*
c) Both a and b d) *A. equili*

982. The characteristic finding of *Sporotrichous schenckii* in the Sabouraud's dextrose agar is the appearance of

a) Cottony white colonies b) Dull white fuzzy colonies
c) Yellowish brown colonies d) Black to brown colonies

983. BCG vaccinated calves may become positive result to

a) Culture b) PCR
c) Tuberculin test d) All the above

984. *Brucella abortus* infects the following livestock species

a) Horse b) Goat
c) Cattle d) All the above

985. The cells in the tumor mass of chickens affected with Marek's disease are

a) Lymphoblasts
b) Small lymphocytes
c) Pleomorphic lymphoid cells
d) Reticulo-endothelial cells

986. Nodular lymphatics in horses is caused by the following agent

a) *H. capsulatum* var. *farciminosum*
b) *Burkohlderia mallei*
c) *Sporotrichous schenckii*
d) All the above

987. Epidemic tremor known as avian encephalitis in chickens is caused by

a) Hepato virus b) Picorna virus
c) Rubula virus d) Morbilli virus

988. The important risk factor in the occurrence of tuberculosis in cattle is

a) Overcrowding
b) Extensive management
c) Semi-intensive management
d) Transport

989. Which one of the following is not a coccobacillus?

a) *B. ovis* b) *Haemophilus suis*
c) *Bordetella bronchiseptica* d) *C. jejuni*

990. The source of infection in *Brucella abortus* in cattle is

a) Urine b) Milk
c) Faeces d) All the above

991. Caseous lymphadenitis and arthritis in sheep is caused by
   a) *C. pyogenes* b) *C. pseudotuberculosis*
   c) *S. aureus* d) *Corynebacterium ovis*

992. Bovine milk can act as a source of infection for the following *Brucella species*
   a) *B. abortus* b) *B. melitensis*
   c) *B. suis* d) All the above

993. African swine fever is transmitted by the tick
   a) *R. sanguineus* b) *Argas persicus*
   c) *Ixodes ricinus* d) *Ornithodorus moubata*

994. 'Bottle brush' appearance in gelatin stab culture is characteristic of the disease
   a) Mycoplasmosis b) Listeriosis
   c) Staphylococcosis d) Glanders

995. Flask shaped vesicles in the conidiophores is characteristic of
   a) *Penicillium sp* b) *Pithomyces sp*
   c) *A. fumigatus* d) None of the above

996. The reservoir for bluetongue virus is
   a) Sheep b) Cattle
   c) Vegetation d) Goat

997. 'Roup' in chicken is commonly called as
   a) Egg drop syndrome
   b) Chronic respiratory disease
   c) Metapneumoviral disease
   d) Infectious coryza

998. The property of mycotoxicosis in animals may be
   a) Muatagenic b) Carcinogenic
   c) Teratogenic d) All he above

999. The most susceptible age group for haemorrhagic septicaemia is
   a) < 6 months b) 6 months to 2 years
   c) > 2 years d) Suckling calves

1000. Asteroid bodies or actinomycotic forms in the kidney is indicative of
   a) *Chlamydophila psittaci*
   b) *Aspergillus fumigatus*
   c) *Candida albicans*
   d) *Cryptococcus neoformans*

1001. Turkey rhinotracheitis is caused by
   a) Gallid herpes virus-2
   b) Avian metapneumo virus
   c) Gallid herpes virus-1
   d) Corona virus

1002. The common source of food borne illness due to *Salmonella* in human beings is
   a) Milk
   b) Meat
   c) Both a and b
   d) Faeces

1003. 'Comet' appearance in liquid media is characteristic in the diagnosis of the agent
   a) *Chlamydophila psittaci*
   b) *Ehrlichia phagocytophilum*
   c) *Mycoplsma mycoides* cluster Lc
   d) None of the above

1004. Formation of club bodies or rosettes in actinomycosis are due to
   a) Neutrophils infiltration
   b) CMI response
   c) Antigen- antibody complex
   d) Lymphocytes

1005. Avian mycoplasmosis is caused by
   a) *M. gallisepticum*
   b) *M. synoviae*
   c) Both a and b
   d) *M. meleagridis*

1006. The main principles in the treatment of tetanus are
   a) Antibiotic treatment
   b) Passive immunization
   c) Supportive therapy
   d) All the above

1007. The pathogenic effect of *Brucella* organisms in livestock is
   a) Polyarthritis
   b) Bursitis
   c) Osteomyelitis
   d) All the above

1008. EDS-76 is disease of poultry having the following as the natural host

a) Layer chicken b) Turkey
c) Desi chicken d) Duck

1009. PPLO infection refers to the disease

a) Chronic respiratory disease
b) Infectious synovitis
c) House finch conjunctivitis
d) All the above

1010. Bastard strangles refers to the dissemination of infection to

a) Lungs b) Meninges
c) Both a and b d) Local lymph nodes

1011. The OIE recommended international trade test in the diagnosis of leptospirosis is

a) Macroscopic agglutination test
b) Dark field microscopy
c) Microscopic agglutination test
d) Levaditi's technique

1012. Mycotic pneumonia in birds is caused by

a) *T. gallinae* b) *A. parasiticus*
c) *A. fumigatus* d) All the above

1013. The serotypes of bluetongue virus are

a) 7 b) 10
c) 24 d) 14

1014. The staining technique employed in the diagnosis of Jhone's disease is

a) Modified Z- N technique b) Gram's technique
c) Z-N technique d) LCB staining

1015. 'Inverted fir tree' appearance in gelatin stab culture is characteristic of the disease

a) Swine erysipelas b) Anthrax
c) Both a and b d) Glanders

1016. Anaplasmosis in ruminants is not characterized by

a) Anemia
b) Jaundice
c) Splenomegaly
d) Nephritis

1017. Ovine enzootic abortion is a disease of goats caused by

a) *Chlamydophila abortus*
b) *Brucella melitensis*
c) *Campylobacter foetus venerealis*
d) *Cryptococcus neoformans*

1018. Q fever is caused by *Coxiella burnetti* which is an

a) Intracellular coccus
b) Intracellular bacillus
c) Intracellular coccobacillus
d) Extracellular bacillus

1019. The breed which is highly susceptible for histoplasmosis in dog is

a) Pointer
b) Weimeranner
c) Both a and b
d) Labrador

1020. The pathogenic fimbrial antigen of *E.coli* in piglets is

a) K 88^{+}
b) K 99^{+}
c) H antigen
d) LPS

1021. The characteristic finding of *Histoplasma capsulatum* in the Sabouraud's dextrose agar is the appearance of

a) Cottony white colonies
b) Bluish green colonies
c) Yellowish brown colonies
d) Black to brown colonies

1022. Which one of the following is not a synonym of botulism?

a) Lock jaw
b) Alkali disease
c) Western duck sickness
d) Falling disease

1023. 'Bumble foot' in chicken is caused by

a) *Staphylococcus aureus*
b) *C. pyogenes*
c) *Fusobacterium necrophorum*
d) *Pnemidocopotes mutans*

1024. Heartwater disease in cattle is caused by

a) *Ehrlichia ruminantium*
b) *E. phagocytophilum*
c) *E. bovis*
d) None of the above

1025. The characteristic sign in acute swine erysipelas infection is

a) Pneumonia
b) Rhomboid skin lesions
c) Arthritis
d) Rashes

1026. Intra-follicular and nodular tumours are seen in bursa of chickens affected with

a) Aspergillosis
b) Infectious bursal disease
c) Mycoplasmosis
d) Avian leukosis

1027. Potassium iodide can be the recommended in the treatment of

a) Brooder pneumonia
b) Epizootic lymphangitis
c) Actinomycosis
d) All the above

1028. The drug recommended in the treatment of haemorrhagic septicaemia is

a) Tetracyclines
b) Sulphamethazine
c) Ampicillin
d) None of the above

1029. 'Fried egg' appearance in solid media is characteristic in the diagnosis of the following disease

a) Chlamydophilosis
b) CBPP
c) *B. anthracis*
d) None of the above

1030. The bacteria *Mycobacterium paratuberculosis* can be seen inside the

a) Macrophages
b) Neutrophils
c) Lymphocytes
d) None of the above

1031. In cattle, cold mastitis is usually caused by

a) *Arcanobacter pyogenes*
b) *P. haemolytica*
c) *Cryptococcus neoformans*
d) *Leptospira* Hardjo

1032. The pathogenic effects of aspergillosis in birds is

a) Nodular lungs
b) Bronchopneumonia
c) Vasculitis and thrombus formation
d) All the above

1033. The predilection site of *Brucella* organisms in livestock is

a) Joints
b) Lymph nodes
c) Genital tract
d) All the above

1034. The OIE recommended confirmatory test in the diagnosis of CCPP is

a) CFT
b) Agglutination test
c) CIEP
d) Growth inhibition test

1035. Heartwater disease in ruminants is primarily transmitted by

a) *Amblyomma sp.*
b) *Dermacenter sp*
c) *Ixodes sp*
d) Biting midges

1036. Which one of the following is the common clinical form of infectious bronchitis?

a) Reproductive form
b) Respiratory form
c) Uraemic form
d) All the above

1037. Coomb's test is generally useful in the diagnosis of brucellosis in

a) Cattle
b) Sheep
c) Human
d) All the above

1038. The common cause of bovine mastitis which has zoonotic importance in dairy products is

a) *Streptococcus agalactiae*
b) *E.coli*
c) *Staphylococcus aureus*
d) *Streptococcus uberis*

1039. 'Boot-like' appearance of long bones in chicken is characteristic of the disease

a) Marek's disease
b) Chicken infectious anaemia
c) Lymphoid leukosis
d) None of the above

1040. The cause of death in anthrax cases is

a) Renal failure
b) Shock
c) Both a and b
d) Splenomegaly

1041. Infectious bronchitis is a viral disease of economic significance in

a) Layer chicken
b) Broiler chicken
c) Turkeys
d) Grower chicken

1042. The infective stage of *D. congolensis* is

a) Zoospores
b) Microconidia
c) Conidiospores
d) Arthrospores

1043. Pulmonary and intestinal form of anthrax are common in

a) Cattle b) Sheep
c) Human d) Pig

1044. 'Laddering' of gram positive cocci is the microscopic appearance of

a) Actinomyces bovis b) *Streptococcus pneumoniae*
c) *Dermatophilus congolensis* d) None of the above

1045. In cattle, summer mastitis is usually caused by

a) *Arcanobacter pyogenes* b) *E.coli*
c) *Staphylococcus aureus* d) *Leptospira* Pomona

1046. Nasal aspergillosis is common in the following host

a) Dog b) Chicken
c) Horse d) Cattle

1047. The common route of transmission in animal salmonellosis is

a) Oral b) Respiratory
c) Both a and b d) Congenital

1048. The drug of choice for the elimination of carrier status in leptospirosis of dogs is

a) Streptomycin b) Procaine penicillin
c) Doxycycline d) Amoxyxillin

1049. *Listeria sp* are commensals which habitat in

a) Buccal mucosa b) Stomach
c) Nasopharynx d) Teeth

1050. Cowdriosis can be best diagnosed by microscopic examination of

a) Faecal smears b) Blood smears
c) Brain smears d) Lymph node aspirate smear

1051. Which one of the following is not a sign of *Rhinosporidium seeberi* infection in cattle?

a) Epistaxis b) Broncho pneumonia
c) Nasal pyogranuloma d) Rhinorrhea

1052. The sample used for Ascoli test in the diagnosis of anthrax is

a) Serum b) Hide
c) Faeces d) Milk

1053. The colonial character of *Aspergillus fumigatus* in culture is
   a) Velvetty to floccose bluish green colonies in Sabouraud's agar
   b) Velvetty to floccose bluish green colonies in Blood agar
   c) Velvetty or floccose pink colonies in Sabouraud's agar
   d) Cottony white colonies in Sabouraud's agar

1054. Snoring sound in strangles is due to the inflammation of the following
   a) Nasal septum
   b) Bronchial lymphnode
   c) Larynx
   d) Pharynx

1055. The pathogenic fimbrial antigens of *E.coli* in calves is
   a) K 88^{+}
   b) K 99^{+}
   c) O antigen
   d) LPS

1056. Anthrax bacilli can remain viable in the buried carcass for
   a) 1 day
   b) 3 days
   c) 30 days
   d) 30 years

1057. The cow side test in the diagnosis of CBPP is
   a) CFT
   b) Agglutination test
   c) AGID
   d) ELISA

1058. Mastitis is characterized by the following changes in the mammary gland
   a) Physical
   b) Chemical
   c) Pathological
   d) All the above

1059. Q- fever or abattoir fever in cattle is not transmitted by
   a) Inhalation of amniotic fluid
   b) Congenital mode
   c) Inhalation of nasal droplets
   d) Sexual mode

1060. The organ not commonly affected with the avian leukosis sarcoma complex is
   a) Liver
   b) Bursa of fabricious
   c) Spleen
   d) Lung

1061. 'Strawberry- like polyps' in the nasal cavity is characteristic of the disease caused by
   a) *Rhinosporidium seeberi*
   b) *Burkholderia mallei*
   c) *Actinomyces bovis*
   d) *Aspergillus fumigatus*

1062. Which one of the following *Salmonella* serotype is non-motile?

a) S. Pullorum
b) S. Typhimurium
c) S. Abortus equi
d) S. Dublin

1063. The most common form of *E.coli* reported in the outbreaks of enteritis in neonates is

a) Entertoxigenic
b) Enerohaemorrhagic
c) Verotoxigenic
d) Necrotoxigenic

1064. Which one of the following is a risk factor involved in occurrence of infectious bronchitis?

a) Intercurrent infection
b) Male, heavy breeds
c) Cold season
d) All the above

1065. 'Tick fever' in cattle is caused by

a) *Anaplasma marginale*
b) *A. centrale*
c) Both a and b
d) *Ehrlichia bovis*

1066. The reservoir for Q fever is

a) Rodents
b) Stray cats
c) Rabbits
d) All the above

1067. Ringworm like lesions in the foetus are observed in the

a) *Brucella melitensis*
b) *C. foetus*
c) *Listeria monocytogenes*
d) *Aspergillus fumigatus*

1068. Struck in adult sheep is caused by

a) *Clostridium perfringens* type B
b) *C. perfringens* type C
c) *C. perfringens* type A
d) *C. perfringens* type D

1069. The diagnostic stage of *Sporotrichous schenckii* is

a) Oval yeast cells
b) Cigar like yeast cells
c) Microconodia
d) Sporongia

1070. *Dermatophilus congolensis* infection in sheep results in the following

a) Emaciation
b) Loss of wool
c) Lameness
d) All the above

1071. *Borrelia burgdorferi* in chicken is commonly transmitted by

a) *Ixodes dammini* b) *I. pacificus*
c) *I. persulcatus* d) *Argus persicus*

1072. The method of infection in coccidiodomycosis is

a) Ingestion of spores b) Inhalation of spores
c) Physical contact d) All the above

1073. 'Onion ring' appearance of lymph nodes in sheep is a characteristic lesion in the disease

a) Staphylococcal pyaemia b) Caseous lymphadenitis
c) Maedi-visna d) Pulmonary adenomatosis

1074. *Trichophyton sp* affects the following type of tissues

a) Hair b) Skin
c) Nail d) All the above

1075. Anaplasmosis in ruminants may be transmitted by

a) *Rhipicephalus sp.* b) Biting flies
c) *Boophilus sp.* d) All the above

1076. The postmortem lesions of CBPP are

a) Extended head and abducted elbows
b) Marbled appearance of lungs with widening of interlobular septa
c) Presence of turbid exudate with fibrin clots in the thoracic cavity
d) All the above

1077. Which one of the following is not a source of infection for Q fever?

a) Milk b) Amniotic fluid
c) Placenta d) All the above

1078. Bloody scour in pigs is caused by

a) *Brachyspira hyodysentriae* b) Corona virus
c) Parvo virus d) Vesi virus

1079. Aspergillosis in chicks is commonly transmitted by

a) Inhalation of spores during hatching in the hatcheries
b) Inhalation of spores in the chicken house
c) Congenital transmission
d) All the above

1080. Bluetongue is a viral disease which is specific to

a) Cattle
b) Sheep
c) Buffaloe
d) Goat

1081. The measures of prevention in the occurrence of dermatophilosis is

a) Application of *insecticides* externally frequently used to control biting insects.
b) Keeping the animals *dry* to prevent chronic maceration of the skin.
c) Maintenance of adequate *zinc* levels in the feed of cattle.
d) All the above

1082. Lipopolysaccharide (LPS) is an important virulent factor for the following bacterium

a) *Brucella*
b) *Leptospira*
c) *Salmonella*
d) All the above

1083. Anthrax spores can remain viable in the carcass or soil for

a) 1 year
b) 10 years
c) 20 years
d) 60 years

1084. Sporulation of anthrax organisms occur with greater frequency in soil which is

a) Acidic
b) Porous
c) Sandy
d) Calcareous

1085. Strawberry foot rot in sheep is caused by

a) *C. pyogens*
b) *F. necrophorum*
c) *Dichelobacter nodosus*
d) *Dermatophilus congolensis*

1086. The following organ is commonly affected in swine tuberculosis

a) Cervical lymphnodes
b) Lungs
c) Intestine
d) Mediastinal lymphnodes

1087. Intestinal form of canine parvoviral enteritis is common in the age group of

a) < 6-8 weeks
b) > 6-8 weeks
c) > 3 months
d) < 3 months

1088. The common source of infection for aspergillosis in chicken is

a) Contaminated incubators b) Mouldy hay
c) Eggs d) Litter material

1089. Which one of the following is not commonly involved in the concurrent infection with infectious bronchitis?

a) *Salmonella* Pullorum b) *Mycoplasma gallisepticum*
c) *E.coli* d) Newcastle disease virus

1090. First vaccination against canine parvoviral enteritis is recommended at the age of

a) 6-8 weeks b) 8-10 weeks
c) 3 months d) 10-12 weeks

1091. Contagious bovine pleuropneumonia (CBPP) in cattle is caused by

a) Mycoplasma mycoides var. mycoides Small colony (MmSc)
b) Mycoplasma mycoides var. mycoides Large colony (MmLc)
c) Mycoplasma mycoides var caprae
d) *Mycoplasma capricolam var. capricolam*

1092. Which one of the following is true to the properties of *Clostridium perfringens*?

a) Non-motile & aerotolerant b) Motile and capsulated
c) Motile and anaerobic d) Motile and spore forming

1093. *Dermatophilus congolensis* in horses results in the following

a) Rain scald b) Mud fever
c) Greasy heal d) All the above

1094. 'Morocco leather' appearance of liver is seen in chicken affected with

a) Marek's disease b) Gumbora disease
c) Aflatoxicosis d) Avian leukosis

1095. Case- fatality in lambs affected with overeating disease is

a) 10% b) 50%
c) 70% d) 100%

1096. Lambs are highly susceptible to enterotoxaemia due to the

a) Lack of enzymes in the intestine to inactivate the toxins.

b) Presence of tryspin and chymotrypsin in the GI tract
c) Presence of kappa and lambda to activate the toxins
d) Presence of tapeworms like *Monezia* in the small intestine

1097. Cattle affected by CBPP carry the bacteria in the tissue sequestra and are called

a) Lungers b) Inapparent cariers
c) Passive cariiers d) Active carriers

1098. Which one of the following is not a feature in cardiac form of canine parvoviral enteritis?

a) Hydropericarditis b) Congestive heart failure
c) Pulmonary oedema d) Myocardial fibrosis

1099. The strain commonly used in the vaccination against CBPP is

a) T1/44 b) S45/20
c) T1/14 d) Cotton

1100. The risk factor for the occurrence of braxy in sheep is ingestion of

a) Frozen succulent feed b) Abrasive feed
c) High grain diet d) Lush pasture grass

1101. Allotriophagia is an important risk factor in the following disease

a) BSE b) Anthrax
c) Salmonellosis d) All the above

1102. Which one of the following is a clinical feature of CCPP?

a) Thickened interlobular septa
b) Soft and friable lungs
c) Straw coloured pleural fluid
d) Marbling of lungs

1103. The variant of canine parvoviral enteritis virus is

a) CPV-2a b) CPV-2b
c) CPV-2c d) All the above

1104. Young puppies are highly susceptible to canine parvoviral enteritis than adults because of

a) Active mitotic division and high turn -over of the intestinal cells

b) Parasitic and viral infections in the early stage
c) Absence of enzymes to inactivate the virus in the small intestine
d) All the above

1105. Limber neck is a bacterial disease commonly noticed in the following species

a) Horse b) Chicken
c) Turkey d) Water fowl

1106. *Borrelia burgdorferi* in dog is commonly transmitted by

a) Deer tick b) Lone star tick
c) Ear dog tick d) American dog tick

1107. The serological class of avian leukosis in mature chickens is

a) Viraemia with no antibodies
b) Viraemia with antibodies
c) Antibodies with no viraemia
d) All the above

1108. Which one of the following is not a strain of infectious bronchitis virus?

a) Intermediate type b) Massachusetts
c) Beaudette d) Connecticut

1109. Carrion poisoning in cattle occurs due to the ingestion of

a) *C. botulinum* type C b) *C. botulinum* type B
c) *C. botulinum* type D d) *C. botulinum* type A

1110. The recommended method of control in CBPP is

a) Test and slaughter b) Restriction of movement
c) Disinfection d) Isolation of infected cattle

1111. Canine parvo viral enteritis is commonly transmitted via the following route

a) Faecao-oral b) Respiratory
c) Congenital d) Physical contact

1112. Most of the cases of canine Lyme disease are

a) Clinical b) Subclinical
c) Inapparent d) Per acute

1113. Agglutination tests are useful in the diagnosis of brucellosis only

a) After 1-2 weeks of abortion
b) Immediately after abortion
c) After 2-3 weeks of abortion
d) After 3-4 weeks of abortion

1114. Canine parvoviral enteritis may commonly be predisposed by

a) CPV-1 infection
b) Adeno viral infection
c) Canine corona viral infection
d) Rhino viral infection

1115. Campylobacteriosis which causes abortion in sheep is commonly transmitted by

a) Natural service
b) Artificial insemination
c) Ingestion of contaminated feed
d) Embryo transfer

1116. The virulent factor of *Mycoplasma mycoides var mycoides* Sc affecting the respiratory passage of cattle is

a) Galacton b) LPS
c) OMP d) HSP

1117. Black disease in endemic areas is predisposed mostly by

a) Mosquitoe population b) Fly population
c) Snail population d) Hot and humid weather

1118. The term 'Sea-gull' refers to the shape of the following bacteeria

a) *Actinomyces bovis* b) *Campylobacter foetus*
c) *C. pyogenes* d) *Erysipelothrix insidiosa*

1119. The bacterin vaccine used for immunization against canine borreliosis induces antibodies to the following antigen

a) HSP b) OspA
c) LPS d) Flagella

1120. Infectious bronchitis maybe transmitted by

a) Inhalation b) Ingestion
c) Vertical mode d) All the above

1121. Paracolon disease in poultry is caused by

a) *Salmonella* Enteritidis b) *Salmonella* Arizonae
c) *E.coli* d) *S.* Pullorum

1122. 'Vaccine failure' in case of vaccination against parvoviral enteritis may be due to

a) Interference by maternally derived antibodies in young pups
b) Lack of timely vaccination in pups at the susceptible age
c) Administration of live attenuated parvoviral vaccine
d) All the above

1123. Lumpy wool in sheep is caused by

a) *Dermatophilus congolensis* b) *F. necrophorum*
c) *Dichelobacter nodosus* d) *Staphylococcus aureus*

1124. The common source of infection for aspergillosis in cattle is

a) Contaminated incubators b) Mouldy hay
c) Eggs d) Litter material

1125. The *Borrelia species* which affects poultry is

a) *B. burgdorferi* b) *B. anserina*
c) *B. recurrentis* d) *B. theileri*

1126. Which one of the following is a synonym of histoplasmosis?

a) Cave disease b) Darling's disease
c) Ohio- valley fever d) All the above

1127. Hair perforation test is used in the diagnosis of

a) Dermatophytes b) *Mycoplasma*
c) *Microsporon canis* d) *Trichophyton sp*

1128. Myocardial form of canine parvoviral enteritis is common in the age group of

a) < 6-8 weeks b) > 6-8 weeks
c) > 3 months d) < 3 months

1129. Brooder pneumonia in birds is caused by

a) *Aspergillus nidulens* b) *A. flavus*
c) *A. fumigatus* d) All the above

1130. *Borrelia burgdorferi* in dog is commonly transmitted by

a) *Ixodes dammini*
b) *I. pacificus*
c) *I. persulcatus*
d) All the above

1131. Which one of the following is called valley fever?

a) Leptospirosis
b) Rinderpest
c) Coccidioidosis
d) Equine infectious anaemia

1132. The OIE recommended test in the diagnosis of Lyme disease is

a) FAT
b) ELISA
c) Both a and b
d) CFT

1133. The most common clinical sign of borreliosis in fowls is

a) Meningitis
b) Anaemia
c) Arthritis
d) Biphasic fever

1134. Avian leukosis generally affects chickens at the age group of

a) 7 - 8weeks
b) 5 - 9 months
c) 18 - 20 weeks
d) 50 - 52 weeks

1135. Which one of the following tissue is affected by candidiasis?

a) Cutaneous
b) Mucocutaneous
c) Mucosal
d) All the above

1136. The dose of amphotericin B for fungal infections in livestock is

a) 1.1mg /kg bodyweight
b) 10 mg /kg bodyweight
c) 2.2 mg /kg bodyweight
d) 20 mg /kg bodyweight

1137. The different species of candida can be identified by the colour reaction in

a) CHROMagar
b) Blood agar
c) Sabouraud's dextrose agar
d) Columbia agar

1138. Which one of the following disease is called lung sickness in cattle?

a) Contagious bovine pleuropneumonia
b) Pneumonic pasteurellosis
c) Haemophilosis
d) IBR

1139. Cutaneous streptothricosis is caused by

a) *Dermatophilus congolensis* b) *Erysipelothrix insidiosa*
c) *Actinomyces bovis* d) *Streptococcus pneumoniae*

1140. The host which is commonly affected by Lyme disease is

a) Dog b) Cattle
c) Pig d) Poultry

1141. The vaccine available for immunization against canine Lyme disease is a

a) Live virulent b) Live attenuated
c) Bacterin d) Toxoid

1142. Which one of the following is called 'cat flu'?

a) Canine parvo viral enteritis
b) Feline infectious peritonitis
c) Feline pan leukopenia
d) Catpox

1143. The complication in canine parvoviral enteritis is due to

a) Secondary infection b) Immunosuppression
c) Septicaemia d) All the above

1144. The OIE recommended test in the diagnosis of canine parvoviral enteritis is

a) Electron microscopy b) HA
c) ELISA d) All the above

1145. Corona virus in cats causes the disease

a) Infectious peritonitis b) Pan leukopaenia
c) Cat flu d) All the above

1146. Cowdry type- A inclusion bodies in tissues by histopatholgy can be found in

a) Contagious canine hepatitis
b) Canine distemper
c) Parainfluenza
d) Rabies

1147. 'Blue comb' is a disease in turkeys caused by

a) Corona virus
b) Herpes virus
c) Parvovirus
d) Mastadeno virus

1148. Allergic test can be employed in animals in the diagnosis of infection by

a) *Coccidioides sp* and *Histplasma sp*
b) *Mycobacterium sp*
c) *Brucella sp*
d) All the above

1149. Infectious bronchitis results in high mortality due to it's

a) Hepatotoxicity
b) Neurotoxicity
c) Immunosuppression
d) Nephrotoxicity

1150. Big liver disease in chickens is caused by

a) Retro viridae
b) Alpha herpes virus
c) Avula virus
d) Alpha retro virus

1151. The common risk factor in the causation of dermatophilosis in sheep is

a) Tick infestation
b) Shearing
c) Rain fall
d) All the above

1152. Hepatic abscess in ruminants is commonly caused by

a) *C. pseudotuberculosis*
b) *Fasciola hepatica*
c) *Fusiformis necrophorum*
d) *Staphylococcus aureus*

1153. Which one of the following causes 'bull nose'/necrotic rhinitis' in pigs?

a) *Actinobacillus pleuropneumoniae*
b) *P. multocida* type D
c) *Fusiformis necrophorum*
d) *M. hyopneumonia*

1154. Maedi, a viral disease in sheep is characterized by

a) Progressive pneumonia
b) Long incubation period
c) Chronic course
d) All the above

1155. The dead end host for Japanese encephalitis is

a) Man b) Cattle
c) Both a and b d) Pigs

1156. 'Greasy pig' disease is characterized by

a) Seborrhoeic dermatitis b) Polyarthritis
c) Subcutaneous oedema d) Cutaneous abscess

1157. Which one of the following disease is called pseudostrangles?

a) Ulcerative lymphangitis b) Caseous lymphadenitis
c) Histoplasmosis d) Melioidosis

1158. The hosts involved in the endemic cycle of brain fever are

a) Mosquito- Ardeid birds b) Mosquito- pig
c) Mosquito- Cattle d) Mosquito - Horse

1159. Peste des petits ruminants (PPR) is a viral disease which is specific to

a) Goat b) Cattle
c) Sheep d) All the above

1160. Greasy pig disease is a fatal disease affecting most commonly

a) < 6 months old pigs b) Sucking piglets
c) Adult pigs d) Sows

1161. The hosts involved in the epidemic cycle of brain fever are

a) Mosquitoe- Birds b) Mosquitoe- pig
c) Mosquitoe- Cattle d) Mosquitoe - Horse

1162. The test recommended by OIE in the diagnosis of PPR is

a) Haemagglutination assay b) ELISA
c) CFT d) Immunofluorescence test

1163. Which one of the following is not involved in the etiology of heel abscess in ruminants?

a) *Actinomyces pyogenes* b) *Strongyloides papillosus*
c) *Fusiformis necrophorum* d) *Dichelobacter nodosus*

1164. Udder impetigo in cattle is caused by

a) *Staphylococcus aureus* b) *Streptococcus agalactiae*
c) *Streptococcus uberis* d) Orthopox virus

1165. Goat plague is caused by

a) Morbilli virus
b) Paramyxo virinae
c) Orbi virus
d) Capri pox virus

1166. Impetigo is a disease which is characterized by development of

a) Vesicles
b) Oedema
c) Tumours
d) Lymphadenopathy

1167. The vector responsible for transmission of Japanese encephalitis is

a) *Culex tritaeniorhyncus*
b) *Aedes aegyptis*
c) *Culicoides variipennis*
d) *Culex tarsalis*

1168. Pulmonary adenomatosis in sheep is caused by

a) Type B or D retro virus
b) Morbilli virus
c) Lenti virus
d) Orbi virus

1169. Glasser's disease is a disease of pigs characterized by

a) Chronic dermatitis
b) Polyserositis and arthritis
c) Subcutaneous nodules
d) Cutaneous abscess

1170. Which one of the following disease does not have long incubation period?

a) Jaagsiekte
b) Katta
c) Maedi-visna
d) Scrapie

1171. Which one of the following is not useful in the detection of somatic cells for the diagnosis of subclinical mastitis?

a) Electronic counter
b) Hotis test
c) Newman's staining technique
d) California mastitis test

1172. The amplifier hosts of Japanese encephalitis are

a) Egret birds
b) Man
c) Cattle
d) Pigs

1173. Impetigo is a disease which affects the following species

a) Goats
b) Cattle
c) Pups and kittens
d) All the above

1174. Wheel-barrow test is useful in the diagnosis of the disease

a) Maedi-visna
b) Louping-ill
c) Ovine pulmonary carcinoma
d) Scrapie

1175. Greasy pig disease is caused by

a) *Staphylococcus aureus* b) *Staphylococcus hyicus*
c) *Corynebacterium pyogenes* d) *Haemophilus suis*

1176. Glasser's disease, a bacterial disease is caused by

a) *Haemophilus parasuis* b) *Haemophilus somnus*
c) *Staphylococcus hyicus* d) *Staphylococcus aureus*

1177. The reservoirs of Japanese encephalitis are

a) Ardeid birds b) Rodents
c) Cattle d) Pigs

1178. Enzootic pneumonia in pigs is caused by

a) *Mycoplasma hyopneumonia*
b) *Mycoplasma mycoides*
c) *Actinobacillus pleuropneumoniae*
d) *Haemophilus influenza*

1179. Japanese encephalitis is generally fatal in the following host

a) Pond herons b) Cattle
c) Horse d) Pig

1180. The serological test recommended by OIE in the diagnosis of brain fever is

a) Haemagglutination inhibition assay
b) IgM ELISA
c) Both a and b
d) Immunofluorescence test

1181. Which one of the following disease is called pseudorinderpest?

a) Transmissible gastroenteritis
b) Vesicular stomatitis
c) PPR
d) Bluetongue

1182. Progressive interstitial pneumonia in sheep is caused by

a) Type C oncorna virus
b) Morbilli virus
c) Lenti virus
d) Orbi virus

1183. Which one of the following is called 'driving disease'?

a) Maedi-visna
b) Bluetongue
c) Jaagsiekte
d) Scrapie

1184. Foot-rot in ruminants may be predisposed by the following pathogen

a) *Trichostrongylus colubriformis*
b) *Strongyloides westeri*
c) *Strongyloides papillosus*
d) *Staphylococcus aureus*

1185. The penside test employed in the diagnosis of subclinical mastitis is

a) White side test
b) California mastitis test
c) Wisconsin test
d) Strip cup test

1186. Which one of the following is not involved in the etiology of bush foot in pigs?

a) *Arconobacter pyogenes*
b) *Strongyloides ransomi*
c) *Fusiformis necrophorum*
d) *Staphylococcus aureus*

1187. Sleepy foal disease is caused by the following agent

a) *C. botulinum*
b) *Actinobacillus equuli*
c) *Leptospira* Bratislava
d) *Corynebacterium equi*

1188. Bovine farcy is caused by

a) *Pseudomonas mallei*
b) *Nocardia farcinicus*
c) *Malleomyces pseudomallei*
d) None of the above

1189. 'Big knee' in goats is a symptom noticed in the following disease

a) Caprine arthritis encephalitis (CAE)
b) Caeous arthritis
c) Foot rot
d) Tick pyaemia

1190. Potomac horse fever is a bacterial disease caused by

a) *Ehrlichia risticii*
b) *Ehrlichia equi*
c) *Streptococcus equi*
d) EHV-1

1191. The drug which is most effective in most of the rickettsial infections is

a) Tetracyclines b) Amoxicillin

c) Streptopenicillin d) Sulphamethaxazole

1.d 2.d 3.a 4.a 5.a 6.d 7.a 8.a 9.a 10.d

□□□

Answers

11.c	12.c	13.a	14.a	15.b	16.d	17.c	18.a	19.d	20.d
21.c	22.b	23.d	24.c	25.b	26.d	27.a	28.a	29.a	30.d
31.b	32.c	33.a	34.a	35.a	36.b	37.a	38.a	39.b	40.c
41.b	42.c	43.d	44.d	45.a	46.a	47.d	48.b	49.d	50.d
51.c	52.a	53.c	54.d	55.a	56.b	57.a	58.a	59.d	60.b
61.c	62.b	63.a	64.d	65.b	66.d	67.a	68.c	69.d	70.a
71.a	72.a	73.a	74.b	75.b	76.d	77.a	78.c	79.a	80.a
81.d	82.a	83.b	84.d	85.b	86.a	87.d	88.d	89.a	90.a
91.d	92.a	93.a	94.a	95.a	96.a	97.d	98.b	99.a	100.c
101.b	102.b	103.a	104.a	105.b	106.b	107.a	108.a	109.a	110.c
111.c	112.b	113.a	114.a	115.a	116.a	117.a	118.b	119.a	120.a
121.a	122.a	123.a	124.b	125.a	126.c	127.d	128.d	129.b	130.c
131.c	132.a	133.a	134.a	135.a	136.d	137.a	138.b	139.d	140.a
141.b	142.b	143.b	144.d	145.a	146.a	147.b	148.a	149.a	150.a
151.a	152.a	153.b	154.d	155.a	156.a	157.b	158.b	159.d	160.b
161.a	162.c	163.c	164.b	165.d	166.b	167.c	168.c	169.b	170.d
171.b	172.c	173.c	174.a	175.c	176.b	177.b	178.d	179.d	180.d
181.a	182.c	183.a	184.b	185.b	186.b	187.a	188.c	189.c	190.b
191.a	192.d	193.d	194.b	195.d	196.d	197.a	198.c	199.d	200.d
201.a	202.b	203.c	204.d	205.d	206.d	207.b	208.a	209.c	210.a
211.c	212.c	213.d	214.d	215.c	216.a	217.a	218.a	219.d	220.b
221.a	222.c	223.d	224.b	225.d	226.b	227.d	228.c	229.a	230.a
231.a	232.a	233.d	234.c	235.d	236.d	237.c	238.a	239.d	240.c
241.d	242.c	243.c	244.c	245.a	246.d	247.a	248.a	249.d	250.c
251.a	252.c	253.a	254.d	255.d	256.a	257.a	258.d	259.d	260.a
261.a	262.c	263.b	264.d	265.a	266.d	267.c	268.c	269.a	270.c
271.c	272.a	273.a	274.a	275.c	276.a	277.b	278.b	279.b	280.a
281.c	282.b	283.c	284.d	285.b	286.a	287.a	288.d	289.b	290.c

291.c	292.a	293.a	294.b	295.c	296.a	297.d	298.a	299.c	300.a
301.a	302.d	303.d	304.d	305.c	306.a	307.a	308.b	309.b	310.c
311.a	312.a	313.b	314.a	315.a	316.b	317.b	318.c	319.d	320.d
321.a	322.b	323.c	324.d	325.a	326.a	327.c	328.a	329.a	330.c
331.a	332.a	333.d	334.d	335.d	336.a	337.c	338.a	339.d	340.c
341.c	342.a	343.a	344.d	345.d	346.a	347.d	348.d	349.a	350.d
351.d	352.c	353.a	354.d	355.d	356.d	357.d	358.a	359.a	360.a
361.a	362.a	363.a	364.a	365.a	366.a	367.a	368.a	369.a	370.a
371.a	372.a	373.a	374.d	375.b	376.d	377.d	378.d	379.d	380.d
381.d	382.d	383.d	384.d	385.d	386.d	387.d	388.d	389.b	390.b
391.b	392.b	393.b	394.b	395.b	396.b	397.a	398.a	399.a	400.b
401.a	402.a	403.b	404.b	405.a	406.c	407.a	408.a	409.d	410.c
411.a	412.d	413.c	414.a	415.c	416.a	417.d	418.a	419.d	420.a
421.d	422.a	423.c	424.a	425.b	426.d	427.b	428.b	429.a	430.d
431.d	432.d	433.b	434.a	435.c	436.c	437.c	438.b	439.d	440.b
441.d	442.d	443.d	444.a	445.a	446.a	447.a	448.d	449.d	450.d
451.b	452.b	453.c	454.b	455.d	456.d	457.c	458.b	459.a	460.a
461.b	462.a	463.d	464.b	465.b	466.a	467.a	468.c	469.a	470.c
471.d	472.d	473.d	474.d	475.a	476.a	477.a	478.a	479.c	480.d
481.a	482.b	483.b	484.a	485.a	486.a	487.b	488.b	489.c	490.d
491.a	492.d	493.a	494.a	495.a	496.a	497.b	498.a	499.b	500.a
501.c	502.a	503.d	504.b	505.d	506.d	507.a	508.c	509.a	510.c
511.d	512.c	513.b	514.b	515.a	516.c	517.d	518.a	519.c	520.b
521.d	522.c	523.d	524.a	525.c	526.a	527.d	528.a	529.a	530.b
531.a	532.c	533.a	534.b	535.a	536.b	537.c	538.d	539.a	540.b
541.b	542.b	543.a	544.b	545.a	546.b	547.c	548.a	549.d	550.a
551.c	552.b	553.a	554.a	555.a	556.b	557.d	558.c	559.c	560.d
561.c	562.a	563.a	564.d	565.d	566.d	567.d	568.a	569.c	570.a
571.c	572.a	573.b	574.b	575.a	576.b	577.c	578.a	579.b	580.d
581.b	582.d	583.d	584.a	585.a	586.b	587.a	588.a	589.a	590.d
591.c	592.b	593.d	594.a	595.d	596.b	597.a	598.a	599.c	600.a
601.c	602.d	603.d	604.d	605.a	606.a	607.a	608.d	609.d	610.d
611.d	612.d	613.d	614.b	615.d	616.d	617.d	618.d	619.a	620.c
621.c	622.c	623.c	624.c	625.a	626.b	627.b	628.b	629.c	630.d
631.c	632.d	633.b	634.d	635.a	636.a	637.d	638.d	639.c	640.c
641.c	642.d	643.c	644.c	645.c	646.c	647.a	648.a	649.b	650.a
651.a	652.a	653.a	654.a	655.d	656.d	657.d	658.d	659.a	660.a

661.c 662.c 663.c 664.c 665.d 666.d 667.c 668.c 669.d 670.c
671.a 672.a 673.a 674.a 675.a 676.d 677.c 678.d 679.a 680.a
681.a 682.a 683.d 684.d 685.d 686.b 687.b 688.b 689.a 690.a
691.d 692.d 693.d 694.d 695.b 696.b 697.a 698.a 699.d 700.d
701.d 702.d 703.d 704.d 705.d 706.d 707.b 708.b 709.b 710.c
711.a 712.c 713.c 714.c 715.c 716.c 717.c 718.a 719.b 720.b
721.d 722.b 723.b 724.b 725.c 726.c 727.d 728.c 729.c 730.d
731.c 732.d 733.d 734.d 735.d 736.a 737.d 738.d 739.d 740.d
741.d 742.d 743.a 744.c 745.a 746.a 747.c 748.c 749.a 750.d
751.d 752.d 753.a 754.d 755.d 756.b 757.d 758.c 759.a 760.c
761.d 762.c 763.c 764.c 765.a 766.c 767.b 768.b 769.b 770.d
771.b 772.c 773.c 774.a 775.c 776.c 777.c 778.c 779.a 780.c
781.c 782.a 783.a 784.a 785.a 786.a 787.b 788.c 789.c 790.c
791.c 792.c 793.c 794.d 795.d 796.d 797.c 798.c 799.c 800.c
801.d 802.a 803.d 804.d 805.d 806.c 807.b 808.a 809.b 810.b
811.b 812.c 813.a 814.a 815.c 816.a 817.a 818.a 819.b 820.b
821.d 822.c 823.c 824.c 825.c 826.a 827.d 828.d 829.c 830.d
831.d 832.d 833.c 834.c 835.c 836.a 837.d 838.d 839.d 840.d
841.a 842.d 843.a 844.a 845.a 846.a 847.a 848.a 849.a 850.d
851.a 852.a 853.c 854.c 855.d 856.c 857.a 858.a 859.c 860.c
861.c 862.d 863.a 864.d 865.d 866.d 867.a 868.a 869.d 870.d
871.a 872.a 873.d 874.a 875.a 876.a 877.a 878.c 879.c 880.c
881.c 882.a 883.d 884.a 885.a 886.a 887.a 888.a 889.d 890.d
891.d 892.d 893.b 894.b 895.d 896.d 897.b 898.b 899.d 900.d
901.d 902.b 903.b 904.b 905.b 906.d 907.b 908.a 909.a 910.a
911.b 912.c 913.c 914.c 915.c 916.d 917.d 918.c 919.d 920.c
921.d 922.d 923.d 924.c 925.c 926.c 927.c 928.c 929.c 930.c
931.a 932.c 933.d 934.d 935.b 936.b 937.a 938.a 939.c 940.d
941.d 942.a 943.d 944.c 945.a 946.a 947.a 948.a 949.a 950.a
951.a 952.c 953.c 954.c 955.c 956.a 957.a 958.c 959.b 960.d
961.b 962.b 963.b 964.b 965.c 966.c 967.a 968.d 969.d 970.a
971.a 972.c 973.c 974.d 975.a 976.a 977.d 978.d 979.b 980.a
981.c 982.b 983.c 984.b 985.c 986.d 987.a 988.a 989.d 990.d
991.d 992.d 993.d 994.d 995.c 996.b 997.d 998.d 999.b
1000.b 1001.b 1002.c 1003.c 1004.c 1005.c 1006.d 1007.d 1008.d
1009.d 1010.c 1011.c 1012.c 1013.c 1014.c 1015.c 1016.d 1017.a
1018.c 1019.c 1020.a 1021.a 1022.a 1023.a 1024.a 1025.b 1026.d

1027.d 1028.b 1029.b 1030.a 1031.d 1032.d 1033.d 1034.a 1035.a
1036.b 1037.c 1038.c 1039.c 1040.c 1041.a 1042.a 1043.c 1044.c
1045.a 1046.a 1047.a 1048.c 1049.c 1050.c 1051.b 1052.b 1053.a
1054.b 1055.b 1056.b 1057.b 1058.d 1059.c 1060.d 1061.d 1062.a
1063.a 1064.d 1065.c 1066.d 1067.d 1068.b 1069.b 1070.b 1071.d
1072.b 1073.b 1074.d 1075.d 1076.d 1077.d 1078.a 1079.a 1080.b
1081.d 1082.d 1083.d 1084.d 1085.d 1086.a 1087.b 1088.a 1089.a
1090.a 1091.a 1092.a 1093.d 1094.d 1095.d 1096.a 1097.a 1098.a
1099.a 1100.a 1101.d 1102.a 1103.d 1104.a 1105.d 1106.a 1107.d
1108.a 1109.c 1110.a 1111.c 1112.c 1113.c 1114.c 1115.c 1116.a
1117.c 1118.b 1119.b 1120.d 1121.b 1122.d 1123.a 1124.b 1125.b
1126.d 1127.c 1128.a 1129.d 1130.d 1131.c 1132.c 1133.b 1134.b
1135.b 1136.a 1137.a 1138.a 1139.a 1140.a 1141.c 1142.c 1143.d
1144.d 1145.a 1146.a 1147.a 1148.d 1149.d 1150.d 1151.d 1152.c
1153.c 1154.d 1155.c 1156.a 1157.a 1158.a 1159.a 1160.b 1161.b
1162.b 1163.b 1164.a 1165.a 1166.a 1167.a 1168.a 1169.b 1170.b
1071.b 1072.d 1173.d 1174.c 1175.b 1176.a 1177.a 1178.a 1179.d
1180.c 1181.c 1182.c 1183.c 1184.c 1185.c 1186.b 1187.b 1188.b
1189.a 1190.a 1191.a

□□□

ABOUT THE AUTHOR

Dr. S. Saravanan, M.V.Sc., Ph.D. : The author is qualified in Veterinary Epidemiology and Preventive Medicine who completed his undergraduate and post-graduate studies at Veterinary College and Research Institute (VC & RI), Namakkal and Madras Veterinary College in TamilNadu Veterinary and Animal Sciences University (TANUVAS), Chennai-51, Tamil Nadu. He has been serving as Assistant Professor at the Department of Veterinary Epidemiology and Preventive Medicine at Veterinary College and Research Institute (VC & RI), Namakkal-2 of TamilNadu, with a teaching experience of more than nine years in this Varsity. He, so far, published 30 research articles, fifty five popular articles and a textbook on 'Common Protozuan Diseases in Livestock - A Student's Guide.